# THE MIRACLE OF ESSENTIAL OILS

## Harnessing the Power of Botanicals to Ease Physical, Emotional and Psychological Trauma

Includes:

Jason's Excerpt from *The Battle Within*
About Post-War PTSD

~ ~ ~ ~ ~ ~

Ryan's Practical Workbook:
The Science Behind Pain and Trauma

## RYAN WATSON, M.ED.
## JASON SAPP

Published by Paradigm Press, LLC
paradigmpressllc@gmail.com
paradigmpressshop.com

First Edition

ISBN: 978-1543005981

Editor and Cover Design:
Mary Jo Stresky
The Write MoJo Literary & Research Services
thewritemojo.com

Iraq Photo Credits:
Jason Sapp (except the Twin Towers photo)

Essential Oils Photo Credit:
Jean Paul Chassenet, Dreamstime.com

Jason's Portrait courtesy of his good friends at
sungoldphotography.com

Ryan's Portrait courtesy of Portraits by Tracy at
portraitsbytracy.zenfolio.com

Ryan's anonymous Case Studies are included with his clients'
permission.

Disclaimer:

# DEDICATIONS

*From Ryan...*

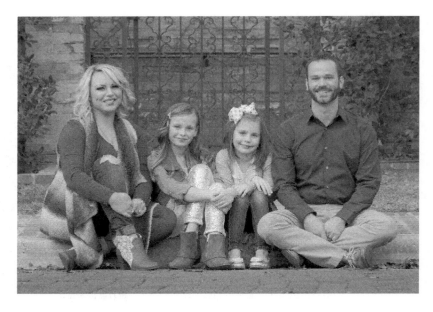

I dedicate this book to my family for their support, encouragement and love throughout the good and bad times in my life.

During the two years it took for Jason and I to compile material to write this book, my wife, Megan, picked up the slack at home, which allowed me the time to get *The Miracle of Essential Oils* finished. I thank her for her direction and understanding, and her fun-loving, humorous personality that kept me focused and on track toward completing my goal.

Above all else, Megan has taught me how to live, has been patient with me, and never left my side while I worked through my own "stuff." From my wife I learned how to have a healthy, imperfect lifestyle in which my family can laugh, cry and enjoy each other more every day. Love you, Meggie!

This book is also dedicated to my two incredible daughters, Natalie and Addison, who told me, "Don't tell us one more time you have to work on the book!" Thank you so much for allowing me to work on my project when I should have been playing Legos or Barbies with you.

I love you for teaching me many life lessons, and how to love more than I knew was possible. I love you both so much!

*From Jason...*

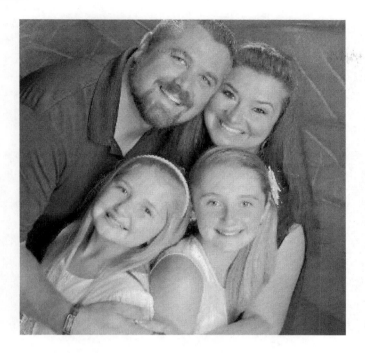

I dedicate this book to my amazing bride, Stephani La'Nette. Her unwavering devotion has been a direct reflection of the unconditional love Jesus Christ has for us full of grace and mercy. I will be forever grateful that you brought His light into my life. I love you, Babe!

I also dedicate this book to my beautiful daughters, Abbygail and Madison. I thank God every day for my two angels He blessed me with. I'm honored to be your dad. I love you both to God and back!

# Contents

# PART III: Bonus Chapter – Sample Tips, Tools and Recipes

## About the Authors (includes contact information)

# AUTHORS' PREFACE

**W**elcome to *The Miracle of Essential Oils*. The material contained within this book is intended to help you holistically take control of your wellness!

At the time they met, Jason Sapp was an Army veteran having returned from service in Iraq. Ryan Watson, M.ED., was (and still is) a licensed counselor specializing in homeopathic approaches to wellness.

During a seminar on essential oils, they discussed why people couldn't get better when using traditional expensive Western medicine that often didn't work.

After they realized they had a mutual passion to spread the word about alternative resources to wellness, they wrote this book to help people think more clearly, have a stronger body, and *live a life of majestic purpose!*

## What You'll Be Learning

Have you wondered if essential oils, and natural, holistic approaches to wellness, can really improve the quality of your life?

### *The answer is a resounding yes, they can!*

Learning about the power and benefits of essential oils is an excellent way to begin your journey to wellness.

You'll learn about the different kinds of essential oils, and their use in overcoming many different kinds of mental, physical and emotional trauma. You'll also learn how to remove toxins and chemicals from your body to return it to a much healthier state.

In his condensed autobiography (more details in his upcoming book, *The Battle Within*), Jason shares the Post-Traumatic Stress Disorder (PTSD) he acquired while serving in Iraq.

He reveals how he used essential oils to overcome the emotional damage that almost destroyed his family and his life.

Ryan's workbook provides...

- background information on neuroscience (the science of the brain).
- tools and techniques to change your body's vibrations, to shift your mindset from negative to positive, and literally tap into your body's awesome powers.
- relaxation methodologies to take you into calmer states.
- ways to remove negative emotion and trauma that block and prevent your healing.
- case studies that show how his clients achieved amazing results by incorporating neuroscience, meditation, affirmations, a healthier lifestyle, and essential oils into their daily regimens.

Collectively, *The Miracle of Essential Oils* contains information for...

- anyone suffering from physical, emotional and spiritual trauma.
- individuals trying to find well-balanced personal and work lives by eliminating stress.
- children and teens suffering from many of the same symptoms and conditions adults experience.
- men and women who've been to war, and experienced stress, hardships and horrific losses in battle and after returning to civilian life.
- individuals working in service-related areas such as firefighters, police and EMTs who suffer from similar kinds of trauma.

A bonus chapter on Tips, Tools and Recipes contains examples of how to incorporate essential oils externally *and* internally into your daily routine.

## How You'll Be Challenged

*"We must look for ways to be an active force in our own lives. We must take charge of our own destinies, design a life of substance, and truly begin to live our dreams."*
~Les Brown

You didn't become unwell overnight, so you can't expect your wellness to occur overnight.

You and only you can take charge of your life and well-being. If you wait for someone else to do it for you, the likelihood is it will take forever or never.

That might sound harsh. But without putting the effort into having a healthy body and mind, you can't feel the happiness, joy, love, peace, contentment and energy you deserve.

Opening the door to your wellness means having the *faith and belief* that something works. Without believing what's discussed in this book can work, you can't walk through the door and leave your trauma(s) behind.

What works for others might not work for you. Because this book presents "alternative" healthier avenues like essential oils, you'll need to remove misconceptions about traditional products and pharmaceuticals that can damage and/or ruin your health.

You might have heard about essential oils, but don't know very much about them. Even if you have, there are always new things to be learned. Challenging yourself to become educated about them will open doors to wellness you never knew existed.

Thank you for having the courage to take control of of your life by joining Ryan and Jason on your journey to wellness. All they ask is that you have faith, belief, and an open mind while reading this book.

## *You are not alone!*

They'd like to encourage you to Like and follow them on their Facebook page at www.facebook.com/paradigmpress, as they'll be providing training events and live Q&As on a regular basis.

Bookmark and check their website www.paradigmpressshop.com – or contact them to be added to their mailing list – to learn about events and speaking engagements.

If you'd like them to speak at one of your events – or have questions about this book's content, or where to purchase additional copies -- you can contact them at paradigmpressllc@gmail.com or www.paradigmpressshop.com for availability and answers.

\* \* \* \* \* \* \*

*NOTE: Before Ryan and Jason discuss how essential oils work in your body, following is Jason's brief accounting of how he beat the debilitating trauma of PTSD. And how he was guided to incorporating the oils into his and his family's life.*

# Jason's Story
## (An Excerpt from his book, *The Battle Within*)

The events I'll be sharing took me on a journey from being a civilian to being in the Army. Then returning to civilian life where I had to kick, scratch and fight my way back to my life.

## Where My Battle Began

After my second tour in Baghdad in 2006-2007, I was honorably discharged and given the designation of a 100% disabled Army combat veteran.

I hadn't been physically wounded (though my back suffered from the weight of the armor and the tasks I did as a gunner, plus I lost some of my hearing). But emotionally it was a completely different story.

Sadly, the VA (Veterans' Administration) wasn't much help. I had placed my trust in the system, but it failed me by not meeting my needs. After I left the service, I tried several times to become involved with the veteran community, but nothing fit the person I had become.

I became trained as a certified veteran peer counselor in Texas. But the group I was part of fell apart after the leaders moved away. I joined the VFW (Veterans of Foreign Wars) and other like-minded organizations. But I realized I couldn't have an impact on the vets like I'd hoped.

In January of 2014, I was first introduced to essential oils because of the damage I had incurred while in Iraq. By that summer, I knew how powerful they were for rebalancing my emotional and physical well-being. So I started researching ways to improve my life without the VA being involved.

I learned I needed to improve my diet by switching to a more organic, whole foods-based diet which made a huge difference in my physical issues. But I knew I needed help with the psychologically damaging wartime experiences as they continued to haunt me.

When I met Ryan at a seminar for the company we purchased our oils from, I knew God had finally opened the door I was to walk through. I initially co-wrote this book with Ryan to reach out to my fellow veterans. However, we now see our goal to changes lives around the world is much bigger than either of us could have imagined.

(Just to be clear, it's not just veterans who can benefit from this book and essential oils. Men, women, teens and children of all ages and walks of life can be blessed with their sacred rejuvenating powers.)

## *I'm living proof that they work!*

With the support of my family, who didn't turn their back on me during my worst times, I emerged from the depths of emotional and physical despair a much better man. I was given a second chance to help people find their way out of the darkness into the light.

The following is a very condensed overview of what happened during my tour of duty in Iraq, and what happened after I returned to the States.

\* \* \* \* \* \* \*

*Some people say they believe in guardian angels, fate or destiny. But I can't look back on how far I've come since my years in the military and not see a pattern of miracles.*

## **Tuesday, September 11, 2001...**

My roommate woke me at 9:00 in the morning, screaming that New York City was under attack by terrorists.

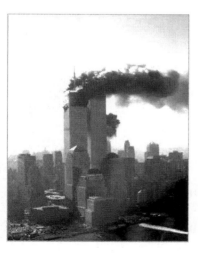

Groggy from sleep, I couldn't understand what he meant until I turned on the television and saw United Airlines Flight 175 hit the second tower at the World Trade Center.

Horrified by what happened, I became desperate to serve my country in some capacity.

So a year later I enlisted in the Army Reserve as an administrative assistant with my goal of going to college via ROTC and become an officer.

In the fall of 2002, while finishing basic and job training, my destiny changed once again when war drums started beating on Saddam Hussein's door.

In February of 2003, my reserve unit called to warn me of a possible mobilization to support Army operations overseas. At the beginning of March, my unit was sent to Ft. Lewis, Washington near Tacoma. Once trained and ready to deploy, I and seventeen of my comrades got our orders to fly out that Monday on an unmarked civilian contract plane to Kuwait.

In the spring of 2004 after my first tour of duty, I requested to have my medical records reviewed in order to have my status changed from reserve to active duty. After re-enlisting on August 8, 2005, I received orders to go to Germany in January to the 1st Infantry Division known as the "Big Red One."

Later that summer, my unit received its orders to deploy. After months of gunnery and urban operations training during the coldest winter in thirty years, we were finally going to the desert.

During the summer of 2006, my first mission in Iraq "outside the wire" was to take two soldiers and join the unit we were relieving in Baghdad. Though I fully expected to take fire while on patrol, I had no way to know how badly it would affect me.

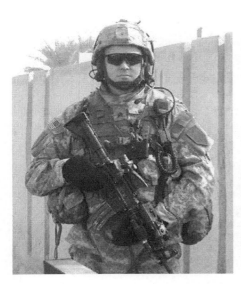

During my time in Baghdad I was shot at and nearly blown up by mortars, rockets and IEDs. I dealt with bloodshed, mutilated bodies, and many horrors I wouldn't wish anyone to hear, see or smell.

The Army does a great job training for combat and the rules of engagement. But there's no way to be trained on what going into actual combat would be like. We also weren't trained to know how to handle surviving while so many were severely wounded or killed. We could only do our best to have a successful mission and get home alive.

Around Christmastime, I began having violent nightmares. Hearing gunfire when there wasn't any, *I knew something was terribly wrong.*

So I went to our brigade mental health team who told me I might need to return to Germany for further evaluation.

I asked to stay until my scheduled R&R in February of 2007. When I met with the mental health officer, he stopped my R&R orders and submitted a recommendation that I should be discharged. Then he began the process of convening a medical review board to see if I was still fit for duty.

While my unit was still in Baghdad, I began the long process to be honorably discharged with a medical separation. What I didn't know was the Army was trying to cover up the exorbitant costs of the war, and the horrendous effects of PTSD on men and women serving their country (including myself), by giving false diagnoses or lower disability ratings than they should have been given.

The Army determined I was to be discharged due to panic disorder **and not PTSD**. Not knowing the difference, I was told that as soon as I got home I'd need to connect with the VA that would give me the proper disability ratings.

Since the Army never admitted I officially had PTSD – and despite having put my life in jeopardy to serve my country – I was separated from the service with a 10% rating and a severance check. (This meant I was denied military medical retirement, and the Army would no longer be connected to me by contract.)

Having read research indicating full-on PTSD symptoms typically takes an additional six to twelve months from the onset of the condition, I realized my escalating anxiety was affecting my daily activities and how I interacted with people, including my family.

The weight of my body armor and gear had compressed three vertebrae into a "C" shape, which the Army couldn't fix. So my doctor gave me a prescription for pain medications.

The psychiatrist I was assigned to put me on a regimen of psychotropic drugs to manage the PTSD symptoms. Counting everything I'd been prescribed, *I was now taking eight different medications throughout a day.*

My PTSD symptoms were becoming stronger and more erratic. Late one evening while driving with my family, we came upon an accident that had stopped traffic on the main highway. When an anxiety attack hit full force, I drove the car up a grassy hill to the frontage road and took an alternate uncongested route.

Later, all I remembered was instinctively turning the steering wheel, putting my foot on the gas pedal, and getting out of there as quickly as possible.

Vivid nightmares became a regular occurrence. Sometimes they'd wake me in the middle of the night. Or my body would react to whatever I was dreaming, which meant hitting or kicking my wife sleeping by my side. Badly impacting my energy, I went to my doctor where I waited for hours, only for him to see me briefly and prescribe more medications.

*My daily drug intake bumped to ten.*

The massive amount of prescriptions, combined with my PTSD symptoms, led to an emotional shutdown that was severely impacting my marriage. Already strained from the lack of quality time at home with my family, I could only deal with with my condition one day at a time.

Having difficulty with my memory, my doctor had me see the VA Traumatic Brain Injury (TBI) doctor in Temple, Texas. After four sessions, I was diagnosed with mild concussion TBI resulting from a mortar attack that had thrown me into the truck's hatch while on patrol in Baghdad. I was prescribed medications to help me sleep, and aid my memory and cognitive functions.

*My daily drug intake bumped to eleven.*

No matter how many times I saw physicians or therapists – or how many prescriptions I was given – there was no answer to my dilemma.

By March of 2008, not only was I experiencing full-blown PTSD and issues from TBI, but nasty side effects from the drugs. In my stupor, I couldn't see the negative effects my symptoms, and cramming as much as possible into a day as a coping mechanism, was having on my family.

*Though I'd left the war behind overseas, my battle on the home front had just begun.*

Emotionally disconnected, fear was the only thing driving me forward. My social worker at the VA said feeling numb was my "new normal," and to "just get used to it."

"Just get used to it."

*Great advice for a wounded soldier, don't you think?*

The amount of PTSD symptoms I was juggling were staggering. Because my medications wore off during the night, I'd wake up the next morning on sheets soaked with sweat. I'd put them in the wash, then map out my day, including the routes to all the places I needed to go.

My high level of situational awareness and constant fight-or-flight anxiety (that Ryan discusses in his workbook) made me physically and mentally exhausted. Having severe trust issues with strangers, I isolated myself as much as possible. On days I felt something was wrong, I went home instead of trying to battle my anxiety.

At night I couldn't shut my mind down. Hearing noises outside, and seeing things through doors and windows that didn't exist, triggered an even greater alertness. My nightmares about war contained real or fabricated situations. For instance, I'd dream of being pinned down by the enemy, while fighting for my life with dead bodies strewn all around me.

I refused counseling, and shut out everyone in my life who cared about me. Sinking into a severe depression, I started drinking while still taking many prescriptions. Though I'd accepted the symptoms as just one more thing to survive each day, I wasn't aware of their signs.

For people with PTSD, depression is the main driver that shuts them down and closes off life. Often masked behind other symptoms, PTSD can be extremely dangerous as it can lead to attempted or successful suicide.

Not everyone with PTSD has the same kind of symptoms. Their experiences cause different reactions. How they react to trauma can affect the level of their symptoms. In other words, my PTSD kept perpetuating itself like a hamster endlessly running around on a wheel.

Some people might have more sensitivity to sights or sounds, while others have more nightmares or anxiety. This is why it can be difficult to properly diagnose PTSD until symptoms have become severe.

In October of 2008, thoughts of dying began to creep into my consciousness. Wanting to leave a world full of pain and suffering, I made my peace with my family (of course, they had no idea of what I was about to do), then took the two bottles of Ambien (about 180 pills) the VA had prematurely sent.

Already feeling the effects of the drug, I dragged myself from the bathroom to the bed. They say animals are sensitive to their owner's conditions. Possibly sensing what I was doing, my black Lab, Jake, crawled in with me while I waited for the end to come.

Not expecting to wake up again because I really wanted to die, I prepared to meet God in the afterlife. I had fully expected to do something right by killing myself that night, and hoped He would understand my desperation to leave my pain behind.

Apparently God had other plans for me as my roommates found me the next morning and called 911 [*my wife, La'Nette, and I were divorced but remarried in 2008 – more about that in my book The Battle Within*].

Once I got to the emergency room, the doctors pumped out about 78 pills, which was enough to save my life. I survived because God knew my life's purpose wasn't over.

Nothing could have prepared me for my recuperation time at the VA in Waco, Texas. All the veterans were on a one-size-fits all medication protocol. Some were given higher dosage amounts than others, and we *never* saw counselors.

On the third day I asked a nurse several times to find a doctor to release me. She said that before I could leave, I'd have to refill all of the prescriptions my doctors had on my list (*can you believe that?*). In order to get out of there, I agreed to their terms and signed the paperwork.

After they filled the prescriptions, I dropped the bottles into a parking lot trashcan and kept walking.

The next few days were extremely rough as I was experiencing withdrawal symptoms. La'Nette, who never left my side from that day forward, noticed that at night I'd stop breathing for a bit of time, then gasp for bursts of air.

After the VA had me do a sleep study to determine I had apnea, they issued a CPAP machine to help me breathe at night. I sounded like Darth Vader breathing heavily while my wife tried to sleep. Although it helped some, most nights I'd unconsciously remove the mask.

Once again I needed something better than what the VA offered for my issues. So my VA psychologist gave me two treatment options: One was a twelve-week in-patient PTSD clinic in Waco, which I quickly dismissed.

The other was an outpatient cognitive behavioral therapy (CBT) program called Prolonged Exposure Therapy (PET) designed to educate people about PTSD and breathing techniques, how to handle anxiety and triggers, and how to use the techniques in real-life situations such as crowds.

*NOTE: In his workbook, Ryan discusses different forms of cognitive therapies such as neurofeedback and tapping to deal with these kinds of traumas.*

The biggest difficulty was retelling the traumatic experiences that caused PTSD in order to help the sufferer realize they were no longer in that situation, and how to process their anxiety and stress to function better. Since I didn't know much about the program, and was unaware of anyone who'd been involved in it, I didn't know how I'd handle it.

The easy-to-learn breathing techniques helped me handle small doses of anxiety during my daily activities. But as you can imagine, I had a much harder time dealing with repeatedly telling my experiences from my time in Baghdad. Reliving the trauma over and over was almost too much to bear.

Each two-hour long session was twice a week for eighteen months. Unable to lower my anxiety level by very much, I learned how to recall my experiences while focusing on something else.

The discussions with my counselor seemed to help, so I learned how to compartmentalize my war experiences into tolerable moments. For example, death and bloodshed needed to be separated from humanitarian missions such as rebuilding schools and helping local markets to stay open.

Because I couldn't go back in time and change them, I was having difficulty managing them in the present. So I had to accept the events for what they were.

PET revealed I was struggling with survivor's guilt because I came home in one piece when many others hadn't. Though I knew it was an issue I had to deal with, I refused further therapy and was dropped from the VA mental health clinic roll once I completed the PET sessions.

Not completely denied all my benefits, every six months I went to the VA out-patient clinic for a routine checkup. One day after a blood draw, the Emergency Room doctor called and told me to get the nearest emergency room as soon as possible for insulin as I could have major complications like passing out or going into a coma.

The battle in Iraq, the battle to get help, and now the battle with my body. Exhausted by it all, I could either give up or trudge forward.

*Like a soldier in the trenches, I chose the latter.*

By 10:30 p.m., my blood sugar was over 490, so they gave me insulin and monitored me for a few hours. After I was released with instructions to see my VA doctor, I was diagnosed with Type II Diabetes.

Prior to my hospital stay, the VA (where I was seeing my doctor with blood draws every six months) hadn't given any advice to help me make changes to my lifestyle and diet to prevent getting full blown type two diabetes (also known as "sugar urine disease" hundreds of years ago).

Not knowledgeable enough about how the body works, I should have been told the signs of diabetes are fast weight gain, frequent urination, drinking a lot of water, anger over being hungry, and general moodiness. I'd been experiencing all the symptoms of diabetes, but didn't know my body was crying out to eat properly.

So now I was also on insulin and a pill for diabetes. My meds had been bumped up so many times, I should have kept the body armor from the war to protect me.

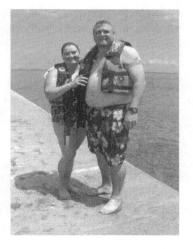

Continuing to wean myself from the other drugs, by the summer of 2011 I'd reached my goal of being off everything except my diabetes medication.

Having a hard time accepting that I'd put on so much weight, I stopped getting on the scale at 298 pounds.

Early fall of that year, I got off the insulin and took just the pill to balance my blood sugar. But that didn't last long, as in December my blood sugar spiked to 400 and they put me back on insulin.

*(The photo is of my wife, La'Nette, and I in Cozumel Mexico in March 2010. This was when I quit getting on the scale.)*

Struggling to find answers, my wife and I both changed our exercise routine and diet, including eliminating most of our red meat consumption. But I was gaining more weight instead of losing it.

Friends recommended that we analyze our diet, start juicing, and eat more veggies and fruits than meat. After watching online documentaries, we still weren't sure how to change our grocery shopping habits.

Honestly, we didn't have a burning desire to do so as it seemed like it would take too much effort, especially after not seeing positive results from our previous efforts.

One day I went into a bookstore and found *The Blood Sugar Solution* by Dr. Mark Hyman who wrote about how dangerous Americans' diets are to their bodies. I read about how to reorganize our kitchen. It even provided recipes to get us started with better eating habits.

Not knowing that organic food was twice the price of the processed food we'd been buying, we made the necessary changes that included juicing and protein shakes to shock our systems into losing weight.

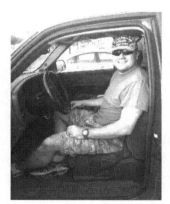

After eight months I'd lost over 80 pounds and was back to my Army weight of 220.

The new diet plan was working! I was now off all prescriptions and insulin for the first time since I was stationed in Germany.

After six long, grueling, painful years, I finally learned a better diet was the key to better health.

*As they say, better late than never!*

Although my overall health dramatically improved, I still suffered from severe back pain.

My bad dreams – as well as anxiety in crowds, and from sounds and smells that triggered thoughts back to the war – were less frequent but still occurring.

Affecting my social life to the point where I had no friends, I knew I wanted that to change as well. But I didn't know where to begin.

Looking to replace allopathic, more mainstream medications with homeopathic remedies, we found several natural options at a health food store for pain such as arnica gel, and elderberry syrup for colds and flu.

In the fall of 2013, we heard about people using essential oils for allergies and other maladies. That concept was completely foreign to me as I assumed an "essential oil" was either thick motor oil or extra virgin olive oil. So I couldn't imagine how it could benefit my body.

The first time I put a drop of peppermint essential oil on my hand, and slowly inhaled the vapors, I was completely floored as I couldn't believe its potency compared to other synthetic ones I had inhaled.

Incorporating essential oils into my daily regimen made me realize how badly educated people are (including myself) about listening to their body's warning signals that something is wrong (Ryan also discusses this in his workbook).

My mind was telling my body that all the processed food and sugary drinks I was consuming was leading to a system malfunction of type II diabetes. So in spite of how far I'd come, I needed to listen to the signals that more healing was in store for me.

The body sends out signals when things aren't going right. While our healthcare system has trained doctors to identify and treat symptoms, many physicians aren't adequately educated to identify system malfunctions.

They might look at a 40-year-old man with a slightly large belly, run blood work to determine if he has high bad cholesterol (LDL) numbers, then prescribe a drug to lower it.

The issue I have with this kind of practice is it ignores the body's warnings. What they might miss is that 40-year-old man might be pre-diabetic, so his body sends signals to his mind that something is wrong. Reacting to a poor diet, his gut has become inflamed. Plus, the high cholesterol is just one of many warnings that something isn't working.

If all he does is take pills for cholesterol, but avoids changing his diet, he'll continue having the same or worse problems. His doctor will continue looking at individual symptoms versus the body's entire system. However, if they paid attention to red flags, and treat the man's body as a whole (holistically), they could prevent further malfunction.

This is just one example of why it's important for you to get to know your body better. You need to become more involved in your wellness. You need to pay attention to signals that indicate something's wrong. After all, who knows better than you what your body is telling you!

It's not rocket science that your diet is a key component to your wellness. You're smart enough to know that when you eat badly you'll gain weight and feel bad. But eating healthy and exercising is one of the simplest precepts that people – including myself – just don't seem to grasp.

Apologies for my digression. But my type II diabetes is a perfect example about the need for an improved diet. Although the doctor had correctly diagnosed my condition, they failed to teach me how to correct my problem outside of prescribing insulin and metformin to "manage" my diabetes.

*Back to using drugs as a panacea – a "magic bullet" to wellness. Now, if that isn't a perfect metaphor, I don't' know what is.*

Though I was taking multiple insulin shots every day, I still drank artificially sweetened sodas. (Hey, I'm a guy. Just like our t-shirts, it's hard to change us overnight.) When I eventually learned that sugar-like chemicals were far worse for my body than actual sugar, I immediately gave them up.

I tried eating less fried food, but still went to fast food places and ate highly processed foods that perpetuated my illness. I'd eat salads, but poured on extra dressing that "drowned" any healthy benefits I'd receive from the leafy greens.

"...a 'healthy' meal is just as susceptible to portion control problems and overloaded add-ons." (For an excellent article on how laden your salads really are with calories, see *How Many Calories Are Actually in Your Salad?* at Huffington Post.) I believed that since our government and food manufacturers had people's best interests at heart, they wouldn't allow bad food to be on store shelves and in restaurants.

*Boy, was I wrong!*

The reality is the majority of them have their own agenda, and don't seem to care about people's overall wellness.

After reading *The Blood Sugar Solution*, I researched what food and supplements the body requires based on the signals it's sending. Learning more about how my body communicates with my mind taught me how to read the signals and symptoms of the parts of the body that need support.

*I've never stopped paying attention.*

## What Essential Oils Have Done for Me

After I incorporated essential oils into my healing regimen, I started seeing a huge improvement in my sleep cycles, my anxiety levels and PTSD triggers, as well as my service-related injuries.

My weight loss, having more energy throughout the day, and my blood work revealed my internal systems were becoming more well-balanced.

The natural ingredients in essential oils release tension, anxiety and stress within minutes when something triggers my mind back to the war. Whereas before using essential oils, it could take days, weeks or even months before I felt relief.

I've also found a sense of peace I never experienced with therapy or allopathic medications. That might sound odd. But in addition to believing the oils work, peace and harmony are the best ways to move your life forward.

It's my firm belief that essential oils should be in the hands of anyone dealing with trauma. For example, people who experience domestic abuse, rape and military sexual trauma (MST) often suffer from trauma and even PTSD.

*NOTE: The different kinds of trauma, and where they show up in the body, are discussed further in the book.*

The earlier essential oils can get into the hands of someone suffering from a physical or psychological condition, the better. People who've been dealing with trauma for long periods of time might be more difficult to reach as they often become secluded, even from their families.

*Never give up on yourself or someone you love, as lives are worth saving! If I could do it, you can as well!*

## You Need to Want to Be Healed for Healing to Occur

The constituents in essential oils are thought to provide relief whether or not a person believes it can happen. For example, a woman uses the oils, but her husband doesn't.

He then gets seasonal allergies and she diffuses lavender oil for him. It provides relief of those symptoms, even if he doesn't believe in the oil's powers, simply because he's breathing in the lavender aroma.

*In other words, his body is smarter than he is because it responds to the oil's chemistry.*

A person *must want to be healed*. They *need to be willing* to work through their trauma, whatever that might be, in order to have lasting, permanent changes. And they *need to believe* essential oils will work so they can have a better quality of life.

Even Jesus knew some people might not want to be healed. In Mark 10:51 He confirmed what the blind man wanted from Him: "And Jesus said to him, 'What do you want me to do for you?' And the blind man said to him, 'Rabbi, let me recover my sight.'" Likewise in John 5:6, "When Jesus saw him lying there and knew that he had already been there a long time, he said to him, 'Do you want to be healed?'"

God has blessed many people with relief and healing from their physical, emotional and spiritual issues. But He won't force it on them because they have freedom of choice. However, with that freedom comes the responsibility to make the right decisions that can lead to their wellness. Otherwise, they'll continue to struggle, and never find a way out of their trauma.

If you want a better life, seek and you shall find it. Don't blindly accept the status quo, or any lack of information and tools, because you can have natural wellness with essential oils. Long-term and permanent healing requires you to want it to happen. Having doubt and no desire to get better only offers temporary benefits from the constituents in essential oils.

Think of it this way: Essential oils are organic compounds made from herbs and plants. Therefore, the oils naturally know how to work in your body. They work for you whether you're awake or asleep, and there are no side effects.

*Can you ask for anything better?*

Most of the vets I met at the VA didn't want to be on medications, especially if it was for the rest of their lives. You'll have to be willing to work out the trauma in your mind. Plus, you'll need to want to find relief to receive the power from essential oils.

*NOTE: In his workbook, Ryan speaks a great deal about the power of belief and faith in order for the oils and treatment protocols to work.*

While reflecting back on the experiences I've shared with you, I've counted the many miracles Jesus has blessed me with over the years. I've found that using essential oils He originally created has allowed me to grow closer to Him.

Through my hardships and obstacles I learned that my life's purpose is to reach as many people as I can to let them know hope and healing is just around the corner.

Trauma can happen to anyone. It doesn't know whether a person's in the military, or if they're a civilian. This just happens to be my story to show you how essential oils brought me back to life.

More than anything I want you to know that...

## *You are _not_ alone!*

The stories and case studies in this book prove that there's light at the end of a very dark tunnel. By overcoming whatever trauma you're experiencing, you too can become a beacon of light guiding others to a peaceful healing.

I encourage you to read the rest of this book, and take charge of your health by doing what's needed to overcome your health issues. Once you find out how amazing this journey to wellness can be, I hope you'll share this book with others who might need it as well.

God bless you for your courage to take control of your life!

## *Jason Sapp*

*NOTE: How to contact Jason and his wife La'Nette about the essential oil program they're involved in can be found in the About the Authors section.*

*Jason's soon to be launched book, The Battle Within, is directed specifically towards men and women in and out of the military. Revealing a full accounting of his experiences while in Iraq, and after he returned to civilian life, will hopefully show them how they can overcome war-induced PTSD and other traumas with essential oils. To get on his contact list to let you know where you can find the book when it's published, send him a note via:*

*sgtjasonsapp@yahoo.com*

*Or get on his email list via:*

*thebattle-within.com*

# PART I

# YOUR GUIDE TO ESSENTIAL OILS
# AND AROMATHERAPY

# Introduction

Your health and wellness isn't to be taken lightly. Learning how to treat conditions and trauma by finding the right products and protocols should be incorporated into your lifestyle.

This means staying with a program instead of quitting once a symptom abates. It means facing your problem, beating it, then keeping it from returning.

Like the blood coursing through your body to keep it functioning, essential oils are the "life blood" of plants that can alter your psychological, physical and spiritual well-being.

Aromatherapy (aroma + therapy) isn't New Age mumbo jumbo; it's pure logic based on actual science. It's a powerful tool to achieving then maintaining a well-balanced life.

Sometimes used as a form of alternative medicine (which is still controversial even in these days of scientific advancement), essential oils complement homeopathy and naturopathy. Plus, research has shown they contain extremely high immune-stimulating properties used to treat many kinds of conditions.

Essential oils are gentle enough for babies, yet strong enough for women, men, boys and girls alike. Because they work from a natural, holistic approach (the whole is more than merely the sum of its parts), they offer hope of wellness during the best and worst of times.

The great news is essential oils are affordable and portable. There's no expensive equipment to use, and no fancy lingo to learn (though Ryan goes into the scientific and medical aspects of essential oils for those who want to learn more).

Once you become familiar with their use, and see their benefits, you'll want them at your fingertips whenever the need arises. Luckily, due to increased awareness of how powerful they really are, essential oils can be accessed online and in stores all around the world.

## The Power in Essential Oils

Have you walked by a plant, bush or tree and inhaled flowering scents like mock orange, magnolia, lavender or lilac? Or have you crushed fresh basil or sage between your fingertips, and salivated at the savory aroma? Or inhaled peppermint or lemon, and all your worries seemed to melt away? What you've experienced is the power contained within essential oils.

## As Old As the Hills

There are over 500 references to essential oils in the Bible, some of which were used for the anointing and healing of the sick. For example, the Three Wise Men brought gifts of gold, frankincense and myrrh to the newborn Christ Child in Bethlehem:

*"On coming to the house, they saw the child with his mother Mary, and they bowed down and worshiped him.
Then they opened their treasures and presented him with gifts of gold, Frankincense and myrrh."*
(Matthew 2:11, New King James Version)

Twenty thousand year-old cave paintings in the Dordogne region of France show plants and their oils being used for medicinal purposes. Even the Egyptians in 4500 B.C. were known to incorporate imported oils from plants that grew along the Nile River into ointments, food, spices, perfumes and skin creams.

Used homeopathically for thousands of years by many cultures around the world, essential oils (also known as "volatile oils") are the fragrance from plants that inspire a positive emotional state, support your physical wellness, purify your home, refine your skin, and create deep spiritual awareness – just to name a few of their many purposes.

The awareness of the benefits of using essential oils and aromatherapy to heal, soothe, calm and abate all sorts of conditions and maladies has become more prevalent over the past decades. For example, businesses around the world are infusing essential oils like lemon and peppermint into the work environment to achieve a calmer, more focused atmosphere:

*"Research by Japanese fragrance company Takasago has shown that staff working in a lavender-scented environment made 20% fewer errors than usual, with this rising to 33% with jasmine oil and 54% with lemon oil.*

*In light of the evidence, the UK branch of Japanese construction company Shimizu now uses scented diffusers to create a productive work environment, as well as creating new buildings with specially designed air ducts for aromatherapy purposes.*

*In its own offices, Shimizu greets workers with a lemon-scented wake-up call, followed by rose fragrance to encourage contentment. The company then combats the post-lunch slump with invigorating cypress smells, and it fills conference rooms with peppermint odors to keep workers alert in meetings.*

*'Aromatherapy is just one of the ways we try to make our workers more comfortable in our offices,' says a Shimizu spokesman. 'It may seem strange to European businesses. But this practice is widely used in Japan, and has been shown to have a positive effect on productivity'."* ("Aromatherapy in the Workplace.")

## Our Core Message

We wrote this book to prepare you for the different stages that occur within your body, mind and spirit when you incorporate essential oils into your daily routine. We also wrote it as a basic guide to understand how essential oils and aromatherapy can support or supersede traditional medical practices.

We're not saying the organic oils we've listed are better than others, or the only ones to use. But it's been found that everyone's body responds differently to synthetic chemicals and homeopathic treatments. So finding a balance between traditional medicine and homeopathy – or using one or the other – needs to be determined to help you know what works and feels best in your body.

Learning how to shift negative vibrations to positive ones might seem like a daunting task, and sound a bit "out there." But if you believe it's possible, it can happen (as Ryan's case studies can attest to).

Our book is a simple comprehensive guide to get you going on your journey to wellness! So why search elsewhere, when everything is literally at your fingertips?

(Mentioning fingertips, Ryan shows you how to use oils with tapping – a truly amazing tool to re-balance and re-center your physical and emotional state!)

We've done our best to provide as much information as possible without overwhelming you. How you utilize it will be up to you.

# Conditions that Can Benefit from Essential Oils And Aromatherapy

## Understanding Your Kind of Trauma

According to the Substance Abuse and Mental Health Services Administration (SAMHSA), there are many different kinds of traumatic events that can impact the behavioral health of individuals, families and communities:

- physical, emotional and sexual abuse, assault or exploitation
- neglect
- bullying
- community-based violence
- psychological maltreatment
- disasters
- serious accidents
- illnesses
- medical procedures
- victim of, or witness to, domestic or community violence
- historical trauma (that impacts entire communities)
- military trauma
- personal or interpersonal violence (homicide, suicide, other extreme events)
- traumatic grief or separation
- school violence or bullying
- natural or manmade disasters (and subsequent forced displacement)
- system-induced trauma and retraumatization (i.e., abrupt removal from the home, or a sibling separation, sometimes with the use of force, restraint or seclusion)
- terrorism, war or political violence

It can be difficult to identify every type of emotion people suffer from due to trauma.

But before you can address how to heal whatever trauma or issues you're dealing with, you need to first identify what they are.

In addition to the conditions listed above, following is a list of the most common feelings that need to be cleared before you can fully heal. (Some will stick out more than others, so begin with those you feel are more important for your recuperation.):

- abandonment, addiction, aggression, anger, anxiety, approval
- bitterness, blame, bondage
- cellular memory, change, confinement, confusion, control, criticism
- defeat, denial, dependence, depression, despair, detachment, disappointment, disconnectedness, discouragement, disillusionment, doom, doubt, drained
- embarrassed, emptiness, exhaustion
- failure, faith (lack of), fatigue, fear, frustration, feeling lost or alone
- giving up or giving in, grief, guilt
- hatred, helplessness, hopelessness
- I can't, inadaptability, inadequate, injustice, intimacy, irritation, isolation
- (feeling) left behind, limited, loneliness, loss of self
- oppression, overwhelmed
- panic, powerless, pride
- rage, rejection, resentment, resistance
- sadness, scared, self-blame, self-esteem, shame, stress, stuck
- tired, trapped, trauma
- unappreciated, unimportant, unsupported, unworthy, useless
- unfair
- worthlessness

There's no one-size-fits-all approach to overcoming trauma. So you should understand the different types of issues and their causes before you can choose an essential oil and/or methods of treatment. This can be as basic as food or environmental allergies, all the way to suffering at the hands of a bully.

*NOTE: Before you begin your journey to healing, it's always a good idea to have a mental/healthcare professional assess then monitor your issues and subsequent progress. Overcoming trauma can be difficult, so it's best not to do it alone.*

## What Exactly is PTSD?

"An estimated 7.8% of Americans will experience PTSD at some point in their lives, with women (10.4%) twice as likely as men (5%) to develop PTSD." (Post Traumatic Stress Disorder, Nebraska Department of Veteran's Affairs).

Post-Traumatic Stress Disorder (PTSD) is difficult to diagnose and treat because an individual can be experiencing one or more of the following:

- isolation issues
- emotional turmoil
- quick to irritation, anger and rage
- daydreaming about past events
- nightmares
- flashbacks
- physical and psychological stressors
- avoidance of places, things, smells, people, etc., that can trigger flashbacks or a defense mode
- easily distracted and lack of concentration
- paranoia

PTSD dates as far back as the Civil War, though the symptoms have always existed as a result of war or other types of trauma. Initially coined as a term for soldiers suffering from "Soldier's Heart" (shell shock or battle fatigue), the condition was defined by developmental and emotional characteristics of an individual exposed to extreme or life-threatening trauma.

Finally recognizing that it's a bona fide crippling condition, the American Psychiatric Association added PTSD to the third edition of its Diagnostic and Statistical Manual of Mental Disorders, (DSM-III).

*"Posttraumatic stress disorder (PTSD) is a mental disorder that can develop after a person is exposed to a traumatic event, such as sexual assault, warfare, traffic collisions, or other threats on a person's life. Symptoms may include disturbing thoughts, feelings, or dreams related to the events, mental or physical distress to trauma-related cues, attempts to avoid trauma-related cues, alterations in how a person thinks and feels, and increased arousal.*

*These symptoms last for more than a month after the event. Young children are less likely to show distress but instead may express their memories through play. Those with PTSD are at a higher risk of suicide."* (American Psychiatric Association, 2013)

Over the years, Ryan has listened to many of his clients sharing their struggles with PTSD. They talk about the trauma, what it felt like, whether they did or didn't overcome it, and why they came to him for his help (see his workbook for Case Studies).

PTSD can be caused by all forms of abuse to a person's body, their psyche, their emotional state of mind, and even their spiritual well-being.

*The longer they're not addressed, the deeper the damage.*

## Trauma and Underlying Issues

Trauma doesn't know what the person was doing to contract it; it's an emotional response to an event or situation.

The damage from physical and psychological traumas (divorce, work or war-related trauma, alcoholism, sexual and drug addictions, etc.) isn't to be taken lightly. Understanding the brain's neuroanatomy will help you understand behavioral issues.

PTSD and acute stressors can be identified by brain function. For example, functional magnetic resonance imaging (fMRI) demonstrates how blood does or doesn't flow to certain parts of the brain. An EEG, or electroencephalogram, demonstrates the electrical activity of the brain.

Oftentimes the prefrontal cortex, basal ganglia, hippocampus, hypothalamus and amygdala are the main areas of concern. Some of the areas can become over-aroused, while others might be under-aroused. Or there can be any combination of the two.

There are many signatures or indicators a professional like Ryan can often identify. But for the purpose of this book, the overall basic picture is indicated.

Anger or rage often triggers trauma. Learned fear often resides in the amygdala. In order to deal with anger, the brain needs to be balanced between the left and right hemispheres.

With regard to emotions, the left hemisphere is often associated with more positive emotions such as joy, hope, excitement, etc. The right hemisphere is often known for more its negative perspective. (Because the right hemisphere develops first, it's no wonder that habits and cycles are more difficult to break.)

Emotions can also cause the brain to become over- or under-aroused. For example, in Attention Deficit Hyperactivity Disorder (ADHD), the front of the brain is often under-aroused while the back of the brain can be over-aroused. (More about all of this in Ryan's workbook.)

The emotions stated below can serve as a checklist to explore whatever problems might be of concern. Overarousal issues often include...

- anxiety (fear)
- depression
- anger
- aggression
- agitation
- paranoia
- shame
- compulsive behavior
- self-hatred
- suicide plans
- lacking empathy
- exhaustion
- needing to control
- holding grudges

Underarousal issues often include...

- anxiety (worry)
- depression
- helplessness and hopelessness
- irritability
- obsessive thoughts
- being easily hurt
- withdrawing when stressed
- guilt
- thoughts such as "I wish I were dead"
- grumpiness
- lack of self-esteem
- performance anxiety
- rumination
- shyness
- whining
- fidgety
- seasonal affective disorders (SAD)
- jealousy or envy
- listlessness

A psychiatrist (the one that prescibes medication) tries to assess your mental issues so they can prescribe the correct medications. For example, if you're depressed, your brain might have slow activity.

Thus, if your therapist wants to accelerate the activity in different areas of the brain, they would give you a selective serotonin reuptake inhibitor (SSRI) or a similar type of drug.

## Essential Oils Versus Western Medicine

The problem with most prescribed medications is they have side effects that will weaken, dull or even heighten your senses. (Many people report they don't feel connected to themselves, or to God and their spirituality, while taking certain types of medication.)

A study published at the National Center for Biotechnology Information (NCBI looked at how rosemary can increase beta waves (fast frequencies/rhythms associated with normal waking consciousness) in the brain.

Rosemary essential oil stimulates activity in the brain without any side effects like prescription medications might cause. (There are many essential oils that can have a huge impact on the brain. But more research needs to be done before claims on their effectiveness can be made.)

Dr. Terry Friedmann, M.D. (co-founder of the American Holistic Medical Association) conducted a study on 40 children to explore the effects of lavender, vetiver, and cedarwood on their EEGs (Friedmann, Attention Deficit and Hyperactivity Disorder *(ADHD)*). Twenty had been diagnosed with ADD/ADHD, and 20 received no diagnosis.

Several people were dropped from the study due to lack of the ability to follow the study's structure. After 90 days of trying different combinations, Dr. Friedmann deduced that vetiver seemed to be the most effective to support a child having difficulty with attention and distractability.

After the study was completed, many children reported a marked positive change in how they felt, including their performance in school and their behavior.

AIRASE (Association for the International Research of Aromatic Science and Education) conducted a study on the use of over 20 different oils with autisic children at different times for different reasons.

The areas of focus were on appetite, sleep, behavior, focus, anxiety, agitation, gross and fine motor skills. The results in areas of sleep to help daytime function were very impressive. (Other results are posted at Journal of Essential Oil Research.)

Now that you know millions of people suffer from many kinds of issues that might benefit from essential oils, we're going to discuss how your mind and brain control your emotions, and how an unhealthy body can create unhealthy situations.

# Healthy Body, Healthy Life

### *Being healthy is not a spectator sport!*

Becoming educated about alternative methods of healing will empower you with choices. Plus, it will strengthen your belief in what's being taught in this book. So you need to participate in your health and well-being, and quit being a spectator of your life.

## Stop... Listen... Be in Charge of Your Health!

Have you ever had a persistent noise in your vehicle? But your mechanic can't find it, no matter your protestations? Ten doctors might agree on a diagnosis. But will disagree on which treatment modality will be best for their patient.

No one knows your body like you do. Even blood tests can indicate one thing when it can be something else.

People tend to be too focused on symptoms instead of the root cause. Though Ryan's not advocating for you to be your own physician, in a small way he is.

Learn as much as you can about treatment modalities from natural-minded individuals. Trusting your instincts and your body's signals will tell you exactly what you need to do.

For instance, if you go outside into freezing winter air without a jacket, your skin sends a signal that you need protection. Based on those senses you might go back in and get a jacket, or keep going on about your business. The choice about being warm or cold is yours.

## Optimal Health Extends to All Parts of Your Body

Good nutrition is one of today's most controversial topics. There are many books and online resources about the science of food and body functions.

Many people don't understand that every single part of their body, including their teeth, can impact their wellness.

Over the years Ryan had witnessed energetic or biological dentists eliminate all kinds of bad health issues just by improving dental functions. Needing to get specific dental work done, and wanting to get pricing to remove mercury fillings, he searched high and low for the right dentist.

Because he knew his genetic profile (see 23andMe Genetic and Health Analysis below) he knew what was best for his body. Though he isn't experienced in dentistry, he believed it was important the dentist do exactly what he needed done.

Ryan also knew that all of a person's organs' energy (or voltage) is channeled through their teeth (he's not sure why God made humans this way, but he hopes to ask Him one day). If voltage drops in a tooth, the corresponding organ can be affected.

For example, the number two and three upper molars control voltage to your pancreas, stomach and right breast. On the emotional side, they control anxiety, self-punishment, broken power, hate, low self-worth, and obsessions.

(This all might sound a bit crazy. But remember that being educated about your body gives you power over its wellness.)

In Dr. Tennant's book, *Healing is Voltage, Cancer's On/Off Switches: Polarity*, he reports studies measuring the voltage in those two molars. "The most common thing that can flip polarity," he states, "is a dental infection." He also stated that breast cancer often correlates with the same tooth on the same side.

(In his YouTube video, Dr. Ralph Wilson illustrates the teeth and the acumeridians tooth relationship. For more information, you can visit his website at integrativehomeopathy.com.)

Ryan's teeth could have caused him many problems. But because he was educated about the part they play in his body's wellness, he was able to get the correct treatments.

## Your Body's "Infrastructure"

Your teeth are just one example what can go wrong in your body. There are many components to maintaining optimal health, such as a healthy diet and exercise regimen.

Without the right food and good gut health, liver, adrenal, thyroid function and lymph movement, it's difficult for your body to maintain a state high vitality.

Not providing enough natural support for your body's needs, such as proper nutrition, can cause damage to your organs and cellular structure. For example, only taking vitamin B won't support your adrenals alone, as your adrenals also need amino acids, zinc, sodium, and other nutrients to rebuild cells.

Every cell must have everything it needs to function properly then rebuild itself. "If you give the body the nutrients that every single cell needs to work, the body often has the power to heal all of the cells of the body." (Tennant, 2013)

Because different organs need different nutrients, your body needs a good ratio of fats, proteins, minerals, amino acids, electricity, water, and the necessary voltage for the cells to do their work (electricity is discussed in Ryan's Workbook).

If your body is missing electricity or nutrients, then how are they suppose to rebuild? Can you become hydrated if you don't drink water? Questions like these are why a healthy, well-balanced diet is critical while rebuilding your body's infrastructure.

A quick note about water: You might be surprised that not all water is the same. Ryan uses structured ionized water that has a low oxidation-reduction potential (electron donor water, antioxidant water; to learn more on this you can call WPHC to discuss the options Ryan has or can create for your specific needs).

Not only is it a clean, toxin-free water. But it contains structured information (frequencies) and a balanced pH level that hydrates the body more efficiently, which is *very important for people who struggle with chronic trauma or illnesses.*

## A. Healthy Versus Unhealthy Gut

*Trauma and stress are two of the biggest culprits for stomach problems.*

People often have a tendency toward emotional eating or binging during periods of trauma and stress. When someone says, "I have knots in my stomach," do you think they actually have real knots in their stomach? Of course they don't. But the feeling of "knots" is signaling they should pay attention to possible warning signs of stress.

As you'll learn in Ryan's workbook, the fight-or-flight response can alter you body's toxicity. If you have poor detox pathways, such as your liver, then any detox program could be very dangerous. But eliminating the stress that increases the intracellular and intercellular waste issues, proper detox wouldn't be a problem.

Stress causes a lack of homeostasis (discussed later) that leads to problems in other bodily systems such as your stomach. During digestion, proteins break down into amino acids to be used as needed. Therefore, your body needs the right amount of nutrients and energy to help your stomach accomplish this process. However, if your body lacks nutrients that create good sodium bicarbonate, your stomach will struggle with proper digestion. It will digest food for energy instead of rebuilding cells and higher functions that boost vitality.

Greatly affected by what you put into your stomach, gut issues that are often caused by trauma and stress can create issues in other parts of the body. For example, acid reflux is a sign that your gut has become greatly imbalanced.

You need to pay attention to how you feel after you eat certain foods. If you feel bad after you eat, you should change your food selections to see if you feel better. If that doesn't work, something else like diverticulitis or acid reflux might be occurring.

An unhealthy diet means your body spends more energy on digesting food instead of repairing itself. Therefore, high-energy foods are ideal during the healing process. But you want to make sure they contain the right amounts and kinds of nutrients for your body to survive.

One way to determine this is through the 23andMe Genetic and Health Analysis, or the Biological Theory of Ionization (RTBI) which is discussed further in the book. (More information can be found on the Internet. Or you can find out more by contacting Ryan about how he utilizes this method in his practice.)

Early in the healing process, a diet high in good fats like coconut oil, lean protein like almonds, and easily digestible carbs like fruit can be the key to progress. Whereas bad fats (trans and saturated) found in processed food and sugar, certain cooking oils, white flour creates stress on the body as it has to work harder to digest them.

Although good fats are essential for the protective barrier around cells, your body needs rich amino acids (protein) that make up the inner lining of those cells. You can get essential amino acids from healthy food sources such as nuts, seeds, beans, whol soy food, whole grains, vegetables and lean meat.

## Pre- and Probiotics

The human genom project studying human DNA validated that genes aren't as aboundant as previously thought. Some people have weak genetic issues pertaining to the slime layer of the gut. If this is your situation, you need to incorporate prebiotics into your diet to rebuild your gut's microbiota.

*NOTE: While Ryan believes that stress is the main cause of gene weakness, some people might argue with him about that notion. If you're curious about genetic coaching, and what it can do for your health, you can contact him at WPHC.*

Probiotics, such as those found in yogurt and dairy products, are living microorganisms, bacteria and yeast that provide the right environment for food to digest efficiently.

A prebiotic is plant fiber that nourishes healthy bacteria growth in the stomach. Incorporating prebiotics into your diet encourages the growth of good bacteria that combats bad fats and toxins in your gut.

Prebiotics and probiotics work together to create a healthy, well-balanced "ecosystem" as it were in your stomach to help food digest properly.

## B. Your Liver

*If you're nice to your liver, your body will be nice to you!*

A healthy liver supports your immune system, cholesterol production (critical for brain development), bile production, blood cleansing and enzymes.

Your liver creates enzymes that support your gut and all of your organs. Plus, it has numerous functions like creating cholesterol and bile, filtering blood, and other tasks.

## C. Your Adrenal Glands

In *Healing is Voltage*, Dr. Tennant says you can't have longevity if your adrenal glands aren't functioning properly. The adrenals are very sensitive to stress (you'll be learning about fight or flight, and ways to reduce your stress level which will assist your entire endocrine system and other organs to function more efficiently).

A part of the endocrine system, your adrenals are divided into the inner and outer cortexes: One is to help assist with good stomach digestion (which creates more energy from food), while the other regulates cortisol and inflammation.

Affecting alpha and beta receptors in the brain, adrenaline (aka: norepinephrine/epinephrine) alters blood flow to your heart and muscles. The fight-or-flight response boosts energy that causes your heart to race when you feel afraid. (You might have heard stories about cars being lifted off by people who experienced a sudden surge of adrenaline.)

You hear a great deal about cortisol in today's media (especially when related to diet products). Cortisol is a glucocorticoid (steroid hormone) produced from cholesterol (in medication form it's called *hydrocortisone*).

Stress placed on your adrenal glands can cause fatigue, and prevent them from producing cortisol and adrenaline. When this occurs, external stimulants like loud noises, children running and playing, and being asked a lot of questions can become very annoying. The tiniest interruption or stimulant can trigger negative emotions such as anger and frustration.

The body doesn't want to store emotional trauma, so it does its best to operate within homeostasis (your body's desire to maintain internal stability against any situation or stimulus that would disturb its normal condition or function). When your body is out of homeostasis (or "out of sync," as it were) you can experience different types of problems. For example, a racing mind can indicate you're dealing with stress or other issues, which is the body's way of telling you something is out of balance.

## Some Aspects of Your Healing *is* Rocket Science

Any kind of change requires energy. In order to make new cells, your body needs proper nutrients such as water, fats, proteins, carbohydrates, vitamins, minerals and oxygen – all of which you can obtain from a healthy diet.

About 75% of what you perceive as taste is actually from your sense of smell. The taste signal enters the brain through the medulla located at the brain stem. From there it's carried to the thalamus, then the taste centers in the cortex, and then the hypothalamus (that controls hunger and the amygdala (which is discussed in the section on getting a good night's sleep).

Dopamine is a feel-good neurochemical associated with pleasure (no wonder dopamine-containing chocolate is known as comfort food!). Dopamine does other things as well. For instance, you become hungry when dopamine is released into your system. But when dopamine stops, so does your desire to eat.

It's believed that approximately 90% of your body's dopamine is created in your stomach. Therefore, developing the right meal plan to lessen the effects of dopamine can alter the patterns and behaviors for emotional eating.

The balance of all of your neurotransmitters, such as dopamine, serotonin, acetycholine, GABA, and norepenipherine, are important to achieve during your journey to wellness. Implementing a healthy lifestyle is a great place to start.

*Whew!*

Ryan knows that's a lot technical jargon to absorb. But it's important to know that your brain/mind is a very powerful mechanism that controls your behavior and appetite. (He goes into more detail about how the brain and body work together in his workbook.)

## The GMO/Gluten Controversy

GMO means genetically modified organisms. The GMO versus non-GMO controversy is a book within itself. But it's something you need to be aware of while achieving a healthy internal ecosystem.

### Gluten Intolerance

Ryan's father raises corn, cotton, seed maze and other commodities in the Texas Panhandle, Because Ryan has a genetic intolerability for those kinds of foods, he can't eat the wheat raised on his family's farm (wheat consumption is a hot topic in gluten-free diets).

Because the rate of cognitive functions is declining as people age, and Alzheimer's disease and dementia is showing up more and more, could current agricultural trends be the problem with the above-mentioned and other health concerns or gluten issues?

Most people in the agriculture industry would say no, as conventional means are more convenient for the farmer to produce more. Ryan would agree that it does make farming production easier. But is it what's best for you?

There are many factors involved in this complex issue and trend in current agricultural practices. Therefore, it's very important that you become educated on the topic so you can learn what might or might not be best for you.

If you ask any farmer if their chemicals are working as well as they used to or should, or how their soil tests look, many will tell you about the importance of having quality, healthy soil, but that it's difficult to develop and nurture.

Most soil becomes stressed and overworked due to the high demands and competitive means to survive as a farmer in America today. This also affects the quality of the essential oils you purchase as the plants are cultivated in different types of soils with different nutrient levels.

Bioavailability of nutrients in the soil is critical. Modern fertilizers and chemicals don't restore the soil's elements, minerals and other essential nutrient levels, which will affect the brix level (sugar content of an aqueous solution) of the soil, thus the nutrition of the produce. On top of that, add GMO seeds the body has a difficult time recognizing.

All of the above is contributing to the demise of health standards in America. But the "true" cause of gluten intolerance is an age-old controversy.

The microbiota (microorganisms that live in your body) can become compromised from the toxic chemicals used on crops. The toxins will be absorbed by the small intestine, then travel through the vagal nerve straight to your brain. Because you can can't physically feel this occurring, you're not aware of the damage that's being done. More and more people are having issues in this part of their wellness as it often goes undetected.

Americans eat over 130 pounds of wheat per year. Most "normal" blood tests at your doctor's office only include two peptides for gluten or celiac disease. Science has confirmed that there are over 50 peptides, which leaves way too many going untested to determine any sensitivities to gluten and other issues.

Therefore, if you have GMO gluten sensitivities, you'll likely have issues with your gut and brain. With gut issues, your brain can't receive the nutrients it needs to properly function as it requires over one-third of the body's energy supply from food.

So what's the proper way to have gluten sensitivities checked? Oftentimes, an insurance company will only pay for "traditional tests." But there are many naturopathic-minded physicians who have options your insurance might/might not pay for.

Due to the rising awareness of gluten intolerance there's been a massive increase in gluten-free products. So the old days of having an uncomfortable gut are pretty much over.

As we stress throughout this book, the best way to know what's going on is to pay attention to your body's signals. If you eat something containing wheat and you become bloated, and/or have diarrhea, there's a good chance you have gluten intolerance.

## Consume Healthy Non-GMO Food

### Essential Fats

Your brain is composed primarily of fat. Therefore, for good brain power it's important to consume healthy non-processed essential fats.

The book *Nutrition 101: Choose Life!* by authors Debra Raybern, Sera Johnson, and Laura and Karen Hopkins, discusses the differences between saturated, unsaturated, hydrogenated, and trans fats.

They define fats as "...compounds of made up of oxygen, hydrogen, and carbon and belong to a group of substances called lipids." They state that the average American consumes 142 grams of fat per day, when what is really required is only 50 grams or less per day. So no more than one-third of daily fat intake should be saturated fats.

Americans consume too many polyunsaturated and trans fats. Since the foundation of a proper ketogenic diet is healthy fats, you need to consume more good fats than bad. A high-fat, adequate-protein, low-carbohydrate diet, ketogenesis forces the body to burn fats rather than carbohydrates.

A great source of a 'good' fat is extra virgin coconut oil, avocados and butter (no margarine as it's processed oil) and others, as they offer excellent support for your heart, immune system, thyroid and brain.

Just like a squirrel storing away nuts for winter, your body stores fat for colder months. Consuming healthy fats in moderation aids cellular activity that helps maintain ideal health.

When you become stressed, your triglyceride (a fat in your blood that's a major source of energy) levels can rise if your body is in sympathetic lock over long periods of time. (Ryan discusses this and the fight-or-flight response later in the book.) If your body is in a sympathetic lock, your immune and other systems can shut down, causing your body to feel it needs as much energy as possible.

Some fats and simple sugars can be a source of quick energy. Think about the types of "comfort food" you crave (like chocolate that contains dopamine) when you're stressed or anxious. However, consumed in excess can create numerous problems, including a rise in your triglycerides resulting from your liver's inability to break down excess sugar. This can, and often does, cause heart problems if it isn't diagnosed then dealt with.

As it relates to heart issues, stress and proper levels of cholesterol, a mother's breast milk contains 50% of the calories as fat, mainly in the form of saturated fats which are very important for her child's brain development (despite the growing trends by some associations to eat more carbohydrates and less fat).

*Protein*

Besides fats, your body also needs protein. The cytoplasm inside cells is composed of proteins created from amino acids discussed earlier.

In *Healing is Voltage*, Dr. Tennant states, "There are eight amino acids that the body can't make (ten in children). Thus, they are called essential amino acids. To be used, proteins and fats need vitamins and minerals. To date, I have never seen a patient with a chronic disease that is not mineral deficient, and most are vitamin deficient as well."

*Organic Food*

It's difficult to get the proper essential nutrients your body needs if you're not eating well. Many companies add fillers to create less expensive products. So carefully reading labels on cans, jars and boxes will help you become educated about the contents of your food.

According to James Doward's article "Organic Food Back in Vogue as Sales Increase," health food stores and farmers markets have popped up all over the U.S. "After years of falling sales, organic food is making a comeback.

Supermarkets and food associations say that after a sustained decline, demand for organic fruit, vegetables and dairy produce is on the rise, as consumers become more willing to pay a premium for food produced to higher farming standards."

During the summer, a fun activity your family can do together is cultivating a garden, since clean, fresh, organic produce is a terrific source of vitamins and minerals. Vegetables can be frozen or canned without preservatives so you can enjoy them year-round.

## Cleansing the Inside of Your Body for a Healthier Outside

*"Their fruit will be for food, and their lives for healing."*
(Ezekiel 47:12, New King James Version)

Because everyone has specific emotions, genetics, chemistry, etc., there are different physical health concerns to consider. Without an efficiently running digestive system, it's difficult for nutrients to be fully absorbed into your system.

To make sure your stomach is working properly, you might consider doing an internal cleanse (aka: detox). But you first need to make sure your body can handle it. Some individuals need support for basic organ functions, which is very important as a cleanse requires higher levels of energy. So you should consult a nutritionist or dietician or other natural-minded health professionals before beginning any cleanse/detox protocol.

Ryan often discusses beneficial cleanses with his clients. While utilizing a special microscope (the oscilloscope) to understand what plants and animals need for survival, Dr. Carey Reams (ref. RBTI) discovered the many benefits of lemon detoxing to allow the body to ideally function.

A simple lemon cleanse he's done numerous times for his own needs is gentle on the system. Plus, it eliminates many toxins that can cause harm to the body's systems.

Stanley Burroughs, the creator of the Master Cleanse and author of *Healing for the Age of Enlightenment*, discusses the use of lemons, and the art of vitality through reflexes to rejuvenate the body, mind and soul. He mentions effective steps to...

- dissolve or eliminate toxins and congestion.
- cleanse the liver, kidneys and the digestive tract.
- purify the glands and the body's cells.

- eliminate unusable waste and hardened material in the joints and muscles.
- relieve pressure and irritation in the nerves, arteries, and blood vessels.
- build a healthy bloodstream.
- keep youth and elasticity, regardless of your age.

Burroughs created a very specific system on how long you should do this cleanse. Many people have used his methods with great success, and with different results.

(It's a good idea to consult with your doctor or natural healthcare professional before beginning a cleansing program in case you have physical issues that could be exacerbated.)

Burroughs states that you can add the following to your daily regimen several times per day for up to 12 days:

*NOTE: Lemon oil and lemon juice aren't the same. The oil comes from the rind, and the juice from the fruit. Some people might worry that a lemon's pH level is a problem, but you shouldn't be concerned. Although the juice is acid, it's processed as alkaline in the body. However, it could affect your teeth if your calcium levels are low.*

- 2 tablespoons lemon or lime juice (approximately one-half lemon)
- 2 tablespoons genuine grade B maple syrup, preferably organic
- 1/10th teaspoon cayenne pepper
- 1 cup of distilled water only

Ryan uses the following combination:

Juice from 1 whole lemon
1/10th teaspoon cayenne pepper
12 ounces of distilled water

Some people might not need to do this for very long. So once again, you might want to check with your healthcare professional before beginning this type of cleansing/detoxing.

So far you've learned a bit about how your body works, and how traditional medicines can sometimes destroy your system's balance. You've also learned ways to combat ailments by natural means like incorporating essential oils and natural products like lemons into your regimen.

Now we'll go into essential oils and how they work in your body.

# Essential Oils and Your Body

Have you or anyone else in your family ever considered naturopathic remedies for healing a physical or psychological problem or condition?

Have you witnessed someone, or even yourself, using God's natural "medicines"? All you have to do is walk outside to see that His "apothecary" of plants and herbs from which essential oils are made are literally at the tips of your toes and fingers!

## God's Little "Power Plants"

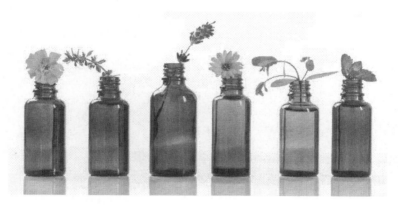

The word oil appears 191 times in the King James Version of the Bible (Stewart, *Healing Oils of the Bible*, 2003) as they were a way of life and well-understood with in those ancient cultures. Using oils for emotional clearing and other religious ceremonies, Egyptians carefully guarded the formulas, such as the following (Stewart, 2003):

- 6 parts frankincense
- 4 parts onycha
- 4 parts myrrh
- 2 parts juniper
- 1 part galanga
- 1 part cinnamon
- 1 part cedarwood
- 4 drops lotus
- 4 drops honey with some raisins

*"As even a casual reader of the Holy Bible might observe, the history of our spiritual ancestors... is one of almost constant motion – migrating and uprooting, shifting from one part of the geography to another.
Indeed, their goings and returnings provide
an incessant rhythm to biblical tales."*
~James A. Duke, Ph.D., author of *Herbs of the Bible: 2,000 Years of Plant Medicine*

A garden is a place of peace, a sanctuary where your body can thrive. The sounds, smells, and sights can take you away from your problems, and help you find balance and harmony.

God created man in the Garden of Eden. Plants grow in a garden aided by sunlight. Since essential oils are from plants, it stands to reason they are "God's medicine" because they contain His healing aromas and light.

Essential oils are made up of numerous compounds that all have a particular job to do. However, not all compounds in essential oils have been identified due to their complexity.

From *Healing Oils of the Bible*, following are "Six Ways that Essential Oils Support Us":

1.  As fighters against unfriendly microbes.
2.  As balancers of bodily function.
3.  As raisers of bodily frequencies.
4.  As antioxidants that purify systems.
5.  As clearers of negative emotional baggage.
6.  As uplifters of spiritual awareness.

You should be pleased to know that essential oils contain only natural, non-genetically modified seeds (GMO).

*NOTE: Jason and Ryan purchase their oils from a provider that distills each plant to retain all beneficial properties post-distillation. Either of them can provide information on how to obtain these 100% therapeutic grade pure essential oils with no fillers or additives, which are much different from what you'll find in health food stores or supermarkets.*

*Their contact information is in About the Authors.*

There are many resources available where you can learn about the chemistry, history and uses of essential oils and aromatherapy (i.e., the *Essential Oils Desk Reference* that can be purchased online is a great start).

From his other book, *Chemistry of Essential Oils*, Dr. Stewart writes, "The chemistry of essential oils consist of simple hydrocarbons, oxygenated hydrocarbons, and their isomers."

Have you heard the term 'carbon footprint'? A life force, carbons are believed to be the most abundant and essential source in the creation of the human heart, brain, and body. Essentially a carbon footprint is greenhouse emissions caused by an organization, event, product or individual.

And yes, that means you as well. Wherever you go and whatever you do leaves a "footprint" in the environment showing that you've been there. So be careful how and where you step!

Over 50 to 70 times more potent than herbs, essential oils are natural aromatic compounds found in the seeds, bark, stems, roots, flowers, and other parts of plants.

Unfortunately, many oils in the marketplace are synthetically created, so they lack any of the organic (and dare we say, healing) properties found in natural extracts. (A clue: real oils come in brown or blue bottles to prevent being compromised, whereas synthetic oils tend to come in clear bottles. Realizing that consumers are becoming more educated about essential oils, manufacturers of synthetic oils are switching to different colored bottles. So you need to make sure that what you're purchasing is a "real" oil.)

Typically, the fragrance and food industries only utilize a tiny, concentrated portion of the oils to make things smell and taste good, so you're not getting adequate benefits from the natural compounds.

The good news is the essential oils we use and discuss in this book are made from the majority of the plants, so you get their full effect!

It's also been found that color therapy can be very beneficial when treating certain conditions. Though carbon can be increased in numerous ways, an easy way is through the color yellow (light). And what better to utilize that light than through photosynthesis (God's "power plant") in the plants and herbs essential oils are derived from.

## Different Kinds of Essential Oils

Though we're grateful for having modern medicine to aid physical maladies, changing negative emotions to positive is key to overcoming many kinds of imbalances.

Thought to be a living organism with a vital life force, essential oils will never force you to do anything you don't want to do.

*NOTE: Though we're listing them individually to educate you about their properties and efficacy, blending them together creates an incredible vibration within your body. Wherever you purchase your oils you should know that due to the fact that essential oils are harvested, they might be in short supply during certain times of the year. Staying in touch about their availability will assure that they're always on hand.*

Essential oils can help you have a long-term, quality life full of peace, tranquility and spirituality. One fun benefit of essential oils is they're portable, so you can take them with you wherever you go to give you instant use and relief.

There's no limit to the time of day or uses for the oils (i.e., while stuck in traffic, at the store with screaming children, in oppressive summer heat, waiting to see your boss for a performance review, helping you to perk up in the morning or during long hours at your desk, etc.).

Many oils can be used topically, aromatically, or ingested. But several oils such as oregano, clove, cinnamon and thyme should be tested first due to their "hot" properties (meaning they can create a hot or warm sensation on the skin.)

"Hot" relates to the viscosity and/or absorption rate. The faster an oil is absorbed, the "hotter" it can become. When you first begin to use essential oils, it's wise to use a carrier oil such as coconut to slow down the viscosity rate.

There are thousands of studies available on research websites on the physical aspects of essential oils. For example, you can visit PubMed.com, then use their internal search engine to find what you're looking for.

Though there are many oils available, following are examples of the most commonly used single-blend oils. As you become familiar with their properties and how they benefit you, you'll be able to determine where they're best utilized.

Then we'll follow that with a list of carrier oils and their booster properties.

## Basil

Eases symptoms of fear or excessive worrying, addiction, adrenal support, general fatigue, and sleeplessness. Because this oil can be an adaptogen for some people (meaning it easily adapts to numerous situations and needs), it can deal with a host of issues. Be careful with its application as it can be "hot" on your skin.

## Bergamot

Eliminates despair, hopelessness, sadness, and weakness. It promotes positive thoughts in order to elevate self-worth. Bergamot was used in early times for relaxation and emotional uplifting. Use this oil when you're feeling down, or during times of stress. Allow yourself to feel relaxed while inhaling its scent to allow all of the aroma to go deep within your body.

## Cedarwood

> *"On the mountain height of Israel I will plant it; and it will bring forth boughs, and bear fruit, and be a majestic **cedar**."*
> (Ezekiel 17:22, New King James Version)

Found numerous times throughout the Bible, cedarwood helps relieve anger, fear, loneliness or isolation. David played his harp made from the cedar trees of Lebanon to help king Saul with his sad mood. The oil has also been thought to empower people by opening their awareness and increasing their courage to change.

## Chamomile (German)

Known for its relaxing effects, chamomile helps decrease stress, and increase clarity, calmness and willingness by stabilizing emotions. It can also aid in clearing negative emotions accumulated from the past. While inhaling the oil, you can use the affirmation, *"I choose clarity for myself and those around me."* (Using affirmations with oils is discussed further in the book.)

## Clary Sage

In the Middle Ages, this oil gained its nickname "clary" as it was thought to help 'clear' eye conditions and hormonal issues. For people desiring to change their negative perceptions, the emotional strength of clary sage helps alleviate confusion, darkness, discouragement and despair.

It's also a wonderful oil for supporting the endocrine system and stress, lifting the senses, helping with bad dreams, and enabling people to better accept their realities.

## Clove

Clove has one of the highest oxygen radical absorbance capacity (ORAC) scales of the single oils, which makes it a terrific aid in wellness care.

Clove oil helps people let go of old patterns of people-pleasing, betrayal, fear, anger, hopelessness, etc. by installing courage and strength. Because it helps relieve negative emotions, it's also a very spiritual oil.

As it's another hot oil, be very careful where you place it on your body (especially keep it away from your eyes).

## Frankincense

> *"And when they were come into the house, they saw the young child with Mary his mother, and fell down, and worshipped him: and when they had opened their treasures, they presented unto him gifts; \gold, and frankincense, and myrrh."*
> (Matthew 2:11, New King James Version)

Found many times throughout the Bible, frankincense is one of Ryan's favorite oils as it encourages openness and awareness while using it with affirmations. You can layer it nicely with other oils.

For example, for relief from negative emotions, first use clove oil with the affirmation, *"I choose to release all negative emotions that no longer serve me,"* then Frankincense with *"I choose to accept joy and happiness."*

Frankincense oil increases your awareness of your truth and purpose, shifts deep-rooted fear to spiritual awareness, and allows opportunity for spiritual growth. Another great affirmation for this oil is *"I choose to accept all that is."*

## Geranium

Geranium is thought to ease nervous tension, lift the spirit, and instill hope and trust. (Two major issues an individual with emotional wounds might struggle with the most are hoping and trusting that everything will work itself out.)

## Helichrysum

This oil helps promote liver function, circulatory issues and skin discomforts by comforting and easing the nervous system. It's known to be very uplifting for issues deep within the mind, and assisting in dealing with despair, frustration and past emotional wounds.

Helichrysum is a high frequency oil, meaning that it's a great uplifter and clears negative emotions. Run this oil from your belly button up to your bottom lip on days when you feel off-balance. Then do the deep breathing exercises, which are discussed later.

## Lavender

Lavender is thought to be the universal oil, as its harmonics are within the frequency range of just about every organ.

Lavender was responsible in part for the resurgence of essential oils by a French chemist after he received a chemical burn. For many years the use of essential oils had pretty much become extinct.

However, "In 1910 French chemist and scholar René-Maurice Gattefossé discovered the virtues of the essential oil of lavender. Gattefossé badly burned his hand during an experiment in a perfumery plant and plunged his hand into the nearest tub of liquid, which just happened to be lavender essential oil. He was later amazed at how quickly his burn healed and with very little scarring. This started a fascination with essential oils and inspired him to experiment with them during the First World War on soldiers in the military hospitals." (Gattefossé and Tisserand, 1993)

Thought by some people to be the mother of all essential oils, lavender is the "oil of expression and understanding" as it's calming. Releasing tension and fear, it helps the user understand the deeper aspects of themselves so they can express their feelings and emotions in a more personal and secure way.

Understanding your emotions opens you to inner freedom, and can prevent you from becoming bogged down.

## Lemon

A terrific emotional and internal cleanser, lemon oil helps promote clarity and concentration, and a sense of safety. It uplifts and encourages, enhances energy, releases tension, decreases mental fatigue. It is a wonderful oil for direction and learning.

## Marjoram

Marjoram is a supportive oil for people dealing with trust issues that can create disconnection from and faithlessness about their life. Isolation can bring on bouts of sadness and displacement, and can escalate thoughts of self-doubt.

## Melissa

Melissa is best known for its ability to awaken and create enlightenment, which is key for mental acuity, creativity, and having a sense of purpose. With people suffering from fear, trauma, sadness, worry, confusion, lack of excitement and joy, and numerous mental health disorders, a decrease in their mental facilities can toss them into a survival mode of just getting through another day. Melissa can be used to positively stimulate the area of the brain that prevents a person from overcoming negative emotions.

Pure therapeutic grade Melissa is often expensive to purchase.

## Nutmeg

Oftentimes with extreme stress or sympathetic overload, the Hypothalamus Pituitary Adrenal Axis (HPA) can become stressed or fatigued. Nutmeg oil can elevate motivation and hope, which helps maximize a person's potential and energy. It's extremely effective when blended with other uplifting oils such as myrrh, peppermint, lemon and others.

## Orange

A citrus oil known as the "oil of joy," studies have found orange oil to be uplifting and relaxing. It decreases sadness and grief, helps people shift their moods by being less rigid and more flexible, and enhances their sense of self-awareness and self-confidence.

## Peppermint

Used to stimulate the mind and body, peppermint oil gets people away from feelings of being overwhelmed and/or sadness. It's known to switch emotional insecurity and negativity to peace and happiness.

Put a few drops of the oil into the palms of your hands. Then cup your hands over your nose and breathe in the vapors to invigorate your senses.

## Pine

When seeking a sense of freedom and relaxation, pine oil has been known to help decrease nervous tension, stress and emotional turbulence. It can energize a person's senses, and brings about excitement and enthusiasm.

## Rose

Said to be the "oil of love," the harmonics of rose oil helps stimulate the high frequencies of the body and brain. And also brings about an emotional, deep healing of the heart. The highest frequency of the oils cited and published, rose oil's frequencies work on the higher senses of self and spirituality by increasing a divine, spiritual connection with God.

## Rosemary

Known since the time of ancient Greece as the "oil of protection," rosemary was burned as incense. Later cultures believed that it warded off devils, a practice that eventually became adopted by the sick who burned rosemary to protect against infection.

Today it's used as for many medicinal purposes such as digestion and indigestion; stomach issues including constipation and bloating; detoxifying the liver and improving circulation, among many others.

## Thyme

Lacking forgiveness increases bitterness, emotional pain, irritation, negativity, anger, and eventually rage. Whereas forgiveness can bring about a sense of emotional entrapment. Therefore, thyme is a great oil for stimulating emotional shifts as it releases trapped emotions, which allows a person to achieve a greater level of emotional freedom and physical energy.

Thyme is also a hot oil, so apply sparingly until familiar with its use.

## Vetiver

Becoming grounded helps people suffering from feeling emotionally torn and disconnected. Vetiver helps decrease stress levels while improving focus, attention and relaxation to create a feeling of centeredness.

Having always had a love affair with Frankincense, vetiver is now Ryan's go-to oil as it has more universal purposes. "Vetiver is an oil I often turn to when acute physical and mental performance is needed, like while writing this book!" he reported. "The combination of vetiver, helichrysum, frankincense, and lavender helps balance my mental washing machine!"

In his 2001 study, Attention Deficit and Hyperactivity Disorder (ADHD), Dr. Terry Friedmann writes about the use of vetiver, and its ability to help with concentration.

## Wintergreen

Wintergreen oil helps loosen rigid thinking patterns by becoming more aware, learning new ways of coping with power and control issues, which allows the brain to shift gears easier, much like you would in a car. It also enhances a person's belief in a Higher Power.

## Ylang Ylang

Known to be the oil of heart connection, love and balance, ylang ylang has an incredible ability to release trauma and stimulate reconnection of self by quietening the mind and quelling negative emotions.

# Carrier Oils

In several of the oils listed above, it was suggested to use a carrier oil to prevent the essential oil from burning your skin. Though essential oils can work by themselves, they're often better enhanced by adding a "carrier oil" to heighten the properties of aromatherapy and the healing aspects of the oil itself.

Known as a "base oil," the plant fats (mainly from nuts or seeds that have healing properties) in carrier oils dilute essential oils so they can be absorbed more efficiently into your skin.

However, diluting the oil doesn't reduce its effectiveness. To the contrary, as it prevents wasting oil because it makes it more absorbable.

Carrier oils can also be used in diffusers (see the bonus Tips, Tools and Recipes chapter later in the book) to elevate an essential oil's aromatherapy properties.

Following are a list of the most common carrier oils to utilize with your essential oils:

## Almond

Almond oil is rich in trace minerals, vitamins A, E and B, and a polyunsaturated fatty acid called linoleic acid. Almond oil's nourishing, softening effects are good for treating skin conditions such as diaper rash, or chafed or chapped skin.

## Apricot Kernel

Apricot kernel oil is a very light oil rich in polyunsaturated fatty acids, which makes it gentle enough to use on sensitive skin and babies. A very nourishing oil, it makes an excellent carrier oil for rashes and dried skin on adults, children and infants.

## Avocado

Avocado oil is the thick, dark green oil derived from the flesh of the avocado. It's particularly rich in vitamins A, D and E, and potassium and lecithin. Avocado oil has excellent healing and skin penetrating properties that makes it perfect to use on dry and flaky skin conditions. It's generally used in combination with other carrier oils.

## Camellia

Camellia oil is recommended for use on the face, and for the healing and minimizing of scars. Camellia oil has excellent hair, nail and skin resurrecting and moisturizing properties.

## Evening Primrose

Evening Primrose oil is particularly useful in the treatment of skin conditions such as psoriasis and eczema, as it's rich in fatty acids such as gamma linolenic acid.

It's recommended that Evening Primrose oil be blended with other carrier oils.

## Hazelnut

Hazelnut oil is excellent for skin penetration and diffusion as it contains trace elements and linoleic acid. Rich in vitamins A, B and E, it's able to penetrate the top layer of your skin without leaving an oily residue.

## Jojoba

Jojoba oil isn't actually an oil as such, but a form of liquid wax which makes it more stable than other carrier oils. Suitable for use on babies and for individuals with sensitive skin, it's excellent for skin conditions such as psoriasis and eczema. It's also an excellent treatment for the hair and scalp. Jojoba can be used on its own, or in combination with other carrier oils.

## Macadamia

Rich in palmitoleic acid that delays cell and skin aging (especially during menopause), macadamia oil is very similar to human sebum. Macadamia oil is soluble, which makes it perfect for blending with other oils. It's also one of the best oils used in skin care products.

## Peach Kernel

Peach kernel oil is high in essential fatty acids. Containing vitamin E, it's wonderful for all skin healing applications, and for use all over your entire body.

## Rosehip

Rich in both Omega-3 and other essential fatty acids, rosehip is an excellent oil for treating conditions such as eczema and psoriasis, and for reducing scarring and healing all skin conditions. Most often used in combination with other carrier oils, rosehip oil can also be used on its own.

## Sunflower Seed

Cold-pressed sunflower seed oil contains essential fatty acids that are particularly beneficial in assisting in all skin healing treatments.

*(Warning: Don't use the refined product found in supermarkets!)*

## Soybean

Soybean oil is light in texture. Containing vitamin E and essential fatty acids makes it ideal for your skin.

## Wheat Germ

Because wheat germ oil is a thick oil with a heavy texture and odor, it's often blended with other carrier oils. Wheat germ oil is the richest natural source of vitamin E, making its skin healing properties ideal.

# Infused Oils

Infused oils are made through the traditional process of cold infusion whereby herbs are immersed in cold-pressed vegetable oils and left to infuse. The oil is then strained, which helps it retain the healing properties of the herbs.

Infused oils can be used on their own, or blended with other carrier and essential oils.

## Arnica

Arnica oil has the ability to reduce swelling, and release and mobilize bruises. It's most beneficial for sprains and strains, and on any soft tissue injury.

## Calendula

Made from marigold flowers, calendula oil is ideal for healing many kinds of skin conditions, including reducing scarring. It's very beneficial for all dry skin conditions, diaper rash, and dry nipples from breast-feeding.

## Hypericum

Hypericum oil is commonly known as St. John's Wort. Used for soft tissue injuries, it's also beneficial for conditions such as neuralgia and shingles where pain is present in the nerve endings.

Now Ryan will take you into his workbook where he'll discuss the basic science of how the mind and body work with essential oils to create a healthy, sustainable life.

PART II

RYAN'S PRACTICAL WORKBOOK:
The Science Behind Pain and Trauma

# An Open Mind is an Educated Mind

*NOTE: In no way is the information I provide intended to treat, diagnosis, prescribe or mitigate your problems. If you feel you have severe medical issues, you should seek the care of a licensed mental/healthcare professional to help you discover, then conquer whatever traumas are haunting you.*

*Please don't be nervous as I'll do my best to walk you through any scientific terminology. But it's really important to understand at least the basics of each of these concepts so you take control of your mental wellness plan.*

One afternoon I received a phone call from a wife whose husband had left the VA. He was ready to end it all because he'd been informed PTSD was the "new normal" for him (much like Jason had been told when he returned from Iraq).

"I just want him back," she wept as she begged for anything to help alleviate his pain and suffering.

Hearing desperation, hurt and pain in her voice, I listened to how her family had been struggling to regain their connection and love they'd had before his diagnosis.

After an intensive session with Bob, he said, "Ryan, I've never slept so soundly. This morning I didn't need coffee as I felt energized and ready to go. I've never felt this good in my entire life!"

Stuck in fight or flight while struggling with stress and emotional trauma, Bob's body hadn't been able to rest. Many people take medications to force their body to change. But their body becomes further imbalanced, which can cause the medication to stop working as well it should.

Because emotions like sadness, joy, anger, etc., are present in the body's tissues, medication dosages are often increased until the person becomes numb. However, facing instead of hiding from trauma helps a person to heal.

I fully believe *skills instead of pills* empower people to live a healthier quality of life. My heart is full of joy and gratitude because the Lord gave me the skills and wisdom to help people like Bob overcome their challenges.

This is just one example of the many phone calls that helped motivate me to build my program. You've made a wise investment in your future, your family and your community by reading this book. I pray the Lord will bless you on your journey to wellness. And that He gives you the joyful ending to your story you deserve!

You might be wondering why I'm discussing the science of the mind and body. The oils work "holistically" with your body's chemistry and nervous system (the whole is more important than the sum of its parts). So it's important to know how your body works so you can understand how the oils bring about physiological changes within your body.

Learning about the science behind what makes the body tick isn't everyone's cup of tea. But because everything I'm discussing is the basis for my work, I felt it important to to show how science of the body and mind work together.

*"The American Medical Association (AMA) has said that if it could find an agent that would pass the blood-brain barrier, they would be able to find cures for ailments such as Lou Gehrig's disease and Parkinson's disease. Such agents already exist and have been available since Biblical times. The agents, of course, are essential oils - particularly those containing the brain oxygenating molecules of sesquiterpenes."* (Stewart, 2003)

God designed your body to be a magnificent, complex, living organism that takes millions of components to run. So it stands to reason that one protocol or holistic application isn't going to work for everyone.

There are many different kinds of modalities, and tools and techniques, available to facilitate change such as...

- aromatherapy (essential oils)
- Biological Theory of Ionization (RTBI)
- cognitive behavioral therapy (CBT)
- emotional release techniques
- energy psychology
- eye movement desensitization and reprocessing (EMDR)
- genetic coaching
- iridology (study of the iris)

- homeopathy
- neurofeedback, biofeedback
- hypnosis
- neurolinguistic reprogramming
- voltage realignment

Because I tend to disagree with statements like "that's just warm and fuzzy," it's my aim to prove these modalities work. The changes you'll experience in your body and brain can be observed and monitored (measured). I'm not saying they're better than other methods. But they're my approach to getting to the same destination, which has fueled my passion for my work.

Most Americans have been traditionally educated about medicine (much of which is outdated). Personally, I wouldn't want to rely solely on a physician trained by institutions supported by the pharmaceutical industry. I'd want them to help me understand more about how my body functions, instead of just writing a prescription and sending me out the door.

The material you're about to learn can be a starting point to shift your mindset from antiquated concepts to ones that meet today's stressful demands. For example, every day I'm learning new, exciting aspects in quantum physics that widen the base of my scientific and spiritual beliefs.

# The Science of Overcoming Pain and Trauma

*(Since I'll be presenting new ways of looking at things, I'd like you to have an open mind while giving them honest consideration. As I said earlier, an open mind is an educated mind. Because I'm a licensed professional, I tend to approach things from a scientific point of view based on tried-and-true methodology. But I've tried to write my material in more layman's terms to help you comprehend it easier.)*

*NOTE: The names of the individuals in the Case Studies have been changed to protect their privacy, and our client confidentiality.*

I received a Masters in Educational Psychology in counseling education from Texas Tech University, a Division 1 university in Lubbock, Texas. Known in the counseling field for its reputation as an outstanding program, the education I received set the stage for me to learn the foundational principles I'd need in my practice.

Over the years my passion for the healing arts grew while witnessing people transform their lives with the modalities I'm discussing (see previous section). I'm fully aware there isn't a one-size-fits-all approach to mental wellness. But I've found the use of aromatherapy and essential oils to be the most beneficial.

The tips, techniques, suggestions and essential oils mentioned throughout this book might not be what you were expecting. But please don't lose faith as you *can* see great benefits from incorporating one or more of them to create a healthier, more well-balanced life mentally, physical and spiritually.

Essential oils changed my and Jason's lives. Frankly, I owe my passion to the work I do to God's garden of medicine-containing plants. But this isn't about us – it's about how the oils can change your lives as well!

## Looking at Your Issues Through New Lenses

You **can** have freedom from trauma and suffering. That might sound great in theory, but not practically if you've tried many things with unsuccessful results.

Throughout the years I've worked with clients experiencing chronic, debilitating emotional, psychological, and physical pain that originated from a perception, an experience, and/or a belief. Most of them have experienced great success because they were willing to try new approaches to their healing. So despite what you currently believe, you *can* shift your paradigm, or the way in which you look, think and feel.

Not only does trauma and PTSD severely affect veterans like Jason, but individuals who have suffered from abusive or traumatic events like the clients I treat through Watson Psychological Health Center in Amarillo Texas (contact information for WPHC in About the Authors), and the individuals who attend the Reconnect and Marriage Intensives.

Combining all the modalities listed in this book over a period of four to seven days can help you become more balanced (integrated) much quicker. Because I often see different stages of healing people go through while they're locked in trauma, integration is very crucial to a well-balanced healing regimen.

There are different levels of trauma I measure to see how much work will need to be done, and what will be the most effective modalities for my clients. My protocol often includes neurofeedback and biofeedback, eye movement desensitization and reprocessing, frequency, light modalities, pattern and movement techniques to work on strengthening neuronal connections, emotional release techniques, and homeopathy that includes aromatherapy and essential oils.

## There is Always Hope!

*"Suicide is the 10th leading cause of death in the United States. According to the Centers for Disease Control, in the United States as of 2010, more people died of suicide than in car accidents. In 2015, the total number of suicide deaths in the United States was 38,364."* (Suicide in the United States; Wikipedia)

Most people know one or more people who committed suicide. Though the statistic 38,364 might not sound high in relation to the entire population, there's no argument that a change in people's mental outlooks is sorely needed.

In my practice, people often say they feel hopeless, that they will never get much better, and that they have to accept or learn to cope with their current state. Through their despair, they feel like they have no choice but to give up and give in. They come to my office as a last resort (which is often the case).

The healing process has different stages. In her book, *Gifts of Imperfection*, American scholar, author and public speaker, Brené Brown, PhD, states that "Spiritual awakening is a process of awareness and acceptance." In other words, just because something doesn't happen overnight doesn't mean it won't work. Your journey to wellness will need prayers, loving and supportive people, and encouragement to prevent you from giving up.

## Shame Resilience 101

Dr. Brown is also a 'shame researcher.' Shame is a key emotion that can keep you locked in numbness, which prevents you from being able to shift into a new paradigm or mindset.

*"Shame is the intensely painful feeling or experience of believing that we are flawed and therefore unworthy of love and belonging."*
~Brené Brown

"Three things you need to know about shame:

1. We all have it. Shame is universal and one of the most primitive human emotions that we experience. The only people who don't experience shame lack the capacity for empathy and human connection.

2. We're all afraid to talk about shame.

3. The less we talk about shame, the more control it has over our lives." (from Dr. Brown's *The Gifts of Imperfection*)

When you make the choice to no longer live numb and hurt, you'll no longer allow your body's vibrations to remain in a gloomy state. So make the choice to open up, and not allow shame be a controlling factor.

You might be thinking that shame isn't a part of your life. But if you think that, it most likely is.

In his book, *A More Excellent Way*, Pastor Henry Wright shares how he was healed by Jesus. Because of that experience, he turned to ministering to others going through difficult times.

Pastor Wright writes that multiple sclerosis is "rooted in deep, deep self-hatred and guilt, and spiritually it is very close to diabetes in that it involves a father's rejection." This is a good example that not dealing with shame can cause physical issues.

I tell people that working on their physical, emotional, and spiritual issues at the same time will accelerate their healing. Your healing will become an inspiration to everyone around you, but it begins with first loving yourself. Then changing your thinking patterns and habits will commit you to taking care of your overall well-being.

Remember, there are several stages of healing people go through. So taking the steps in my workbook will get you on your journey for physical, emotional, psychological and spiritual awakening.

## Smells Trigger Warning Bells

Relating to trauma and aromatherapy, certain smells can trigger positive or negative memories and/or emotions.

*"A number of behavioral studies have demonstrated that smells trigger more vivid emotional memories and are better at inducing that feeling of 'being brought back in time' than images. However, few studies since Herz and colleagues' study have explored the relationship between smell and autobiographical memory at the neural level.*

*Last year, Arshamian and colleagues found evidence to suggest that memories triggered by an odor (like the scent of a rose) were accompanied by greater activity in the limbic system (which includes the hippocampus and amygdala) than memories triggered by the verbal label of that odor (like the word 'rose'). The scientists also found that memories evoked by odors were linked to more brain activity in areas associated with visual vividness."* (Lewis, *Smells Ring Bells*, 2015).

During the early years of my natural approach education, I learned the aroma of an essential oil often relates to a particular emotion or an early life experience. The aromas from oils going through different areas of the brain can trigger stored negative emotions. Sometimes an unpleasant smell can become activated. The good news is the smell can be changed quickly and effectively with affirmations.

## Exercise:
## Using Oils with Affirmations
## to Alter Your Feelings

While at a Center for Aromatherapy Research and Education (CARE) class, I observed the effects of a series of essential oil applications on an individual, and then after connecting them to my mapping equipment. It was astounding to witness actual changes occurring in the different areas of their brain.

Trained to read brain maps, I wouldn't have thought this was possible. Though the results were tremendously fast, overall they were extremely comprehensive on the person's brain activity.

I didn't talk about what I'd seen for quite some time. As I prayed and learned about how God's molecules work in a human's body, I finally understood it was the release of stored emotions. And that the body and brain goes through a chaotic detoxification pattern followed by peace and calmness. (The initial chaotic patterns were difficult to determine as I initially couldn't find any research on this topic.)

For some people the effects of an emotional release might not feel pleasant, while for others it would. Feeling unpleasant doesn't mean the oil didn't work. Rather, it's how a person feels about being normal or safe. Some people have lived with traumatic issues for so long they don't believe they can live any other way. Therefore, the actual state of relaxation would feel foreign and uncomfortable.

Seeing how essential oils can affect the brain had a huge impact on my career by changing my entire approach to mental wellness. A healthy brain empowers people to make changes. The paradigm of talk/thought therapy is shifting as people are learning more about how the brain functions (neuroscience). This scientific revolution is revealing how people can change their thoughts to help themselves.

One of the easiest ways to shift the state of your brain is with essential oils. An aroma has only one synapse to affect the deep emotional center of the brain (the amygdala), as opposed to four, seven, eight or more synapses with another area of the brain.

Once the aroma of an essential oil reaches the amygdala – the part of the brain that helps you deal with problems and trauma – you can quickly achieve a noticeable shift in your emotional and physical states.

However, people who deal with chronic developmental trauma might need to use the oils for a longer period of time before they can accurately determine if they are helping.

Today, more and more professionals are looking to incorporate essential oils into their protocols based on the research of many individuals in the field of holistic medicine.

For example, Dr. Corinne Allen (my mentor and amazing teacher) uses essential oils and affirmations in her program. The following affirmation was a mutual creation of Dr. Allen (in person at the Brain Camp), CARE, and myself:

*"Lord/Higher Self, I ask that you heal every trauma, locked, and blocked*
*cell physically, emotionally and spiritually*
*in all parts of my being."*

First, smell the oil that doesn't smell good to you. Then say the affirmation three times without smelling the oil. Then smell the oil again. This time the oil's aroma should smell different.

If it doesn't, repeat these steps until it does. (I've never seen anyone do this more than three times without having the smell completely change. Many people will enjoy the smell, and want to smell it again.)

If you don't know what emotion(s) need to be released, your unconscious mind will tell you. So pay close attention to how you handle situations from day-to-day. How you perceive them will change over time, and you'll feel more relaxed and calm.

*This is a really cool way to release emotions and feel better!*

# Creating a Life Plan

*"If you always do what you have always done,
then you will always get what you have always got."*
~Author Unknown

Over the years you might have tried to create a structured plan for your life. But certain things, like your emotions, got in the way of understanding then implementing them. For instance, smokers know they shouldn't smoke if they're having lung issues, or a history of cancer in their family. But they keep smoking due to their addiction to nicotine.

People with dangerous substance or sexual predilections know they need to stop to prevent them from ruining their life and other people's lives as well. But they continue to use drugs, or have inappropriate sexual relationships, due to their addiction.

Think of it this way: Why would you need to alter the way you feel if you woke up every morning with a sense of passion and purpose for your day and your life in general? What if you were so healthy that the "high" you felt was life itself?

As a therapist, I could choose many different modalities with the right amount of energy to help my clients during their journey to wellness. But the reason I work with essential oils is there's no other substance on the planet like them. All of the compounds in essential oils have yet to be identified. But the field of aromatherapy is exciting as it offers many magnificent benefits.

Essential oils have chemistry molecules such as *sesquiterpenes* to help reprogram cellular information and many other physical properties. Just as you can release information from the body, you can also cleanse, neutralize, and restore bodily functions.

Essential oils have different levels of frequency, ranging from 320 (rose, *Rosa Damascena*) to 52 MHz (basil, *Ocimum basilicum*). (Stewart, 2003) The higher the frequency, the more an oil affects your higher self emotionally and spiritually. The lower the frequency, the more an oil affects your physical body. Some people like to begin with lower frequencies, then work to higher frequencies to prevent overwhelming their body.

The key to overcoming anything is being able to shift your perspective (paradigm). While studying the frequency of essential oils at Washington State University, Bruce Tainio found the frequency of essential oils in their purest form:

*"Tainio also found that the frequencies of the oils are affected by thoughts. Negative thoughts lowered the frequencies of the oils by 12 MHz, while positive thoughts raised them by 10 MHz."* (Stewart, 2003) (More information can be found at http://www.biospiritual-energy-healing.com/vibrational-frequency.html.)

As you shift your paradigm, your vibrational frequency will change you and everything around you. So remember to apply your oils in a gentle, prayerful manner.

## Custom-Tailoring Your Life Plan

Self-regulation and reconditioning creates positive changes. This simply means that by observing your life plan and creating positive thinking skills, the more empowered you'll become.

Your "life plan" includes the following normal stages of change you'll experience. But it's not uncommon to feel different, or even uncomfortable, while going through these kind of changes:

*Physically*

Just so you're aware of the overall goal or progression, physical changes might be the first to occur. For example, I was talking to a friend about how he uses peppermint oil for his headaches because nothing else works as well (he takes a bottle with him everywhere he goes).

The changes might be subtle. You'll begin to notice that you don't get as angry as often. You might continue to get angry, but you won't experience rage as fast or deep. Plus, you'll know how to control it so it doesn't get out of hand.

*Emotionally*

You might begin to see and feel things differently. Originally you might have sensed the negative in a situation and felt the emotions, and chose to either mention it or hold it inside. But now you don't see or sense as many negative things.

For example, a young lady who came to me about sexual abuse reported that certain scents triggered reminders of the event several times throughout the week. And that she occasionally had bad dreams. Together we were able to connect the patterns and flow of situations to the patterns and flow of her thoughts and feelings.

As she begin experimenting with essential oils, she was worried the aromas might trigger negative emotions. But after a while she noticed she wasn't as sensitive to them as she'd previously been. Because she badly wanted the triggers to leave and never return, she was almost unaware of, and greatly relieved, when they finally did.

## Psychologically

Psychological change can alter your entire awareness and perspective, and how to interact with the world around you.

## Spiritually

Then as life begins to take on different shapes and feelings, your perspective will affect and change your spirituality. The more relaxed, calm and clearer you become, you'll see your past experiences in a completely different light.

I often hear people make comments about being mad at God or not loving themselves. These types of thoughts can change how you see your moral and spiritual convictions. For some individuals, their emotional state doesn't affect them, while for others it does.

As I've observed by adding the power of essential oils to my sessions with my clients, you too can experience deep spiritual and moral changes on a level you could have never imagined.

Knowing the kinds of changes and experiences you'll experience during your journey to transformation will be a great advantage. Although they might not be familiar, the "road map" this book provides will help keep you on a straight and narrow path to wellness.

# Fight, Flight or Freeze

*"Insanity is doing the same thing over and over again and expecting a different result."*
~Albert Einstein

Have you watched a horror film where a character freezes in fear when they see a scary shadow approaching them? Have you ever been in a situation where you feel someone is following you, and you have the urge to run? Or you became so paralyzed that your feet couldn't move?

In a nutshell, that's the "fight-or-flight" response (the first example is the sympathetic lock I'll be discussing).

*"The fight-or-flight response is a physiological reaction that occurs in response to a perceived harmful event, attack, or threat to survival. It was first described by Walter Bradford Cannon. His theory states that animals react to threats with a general discharge of the sympathetic nervous system, preparing the animal for fighting or fleeing.*

*More specifically, the adrenal medulla produces a hormonal cascade that results in the secretion of catecholamines, especially norepinephrine and epinephrine. The hormones estrogen, testosterone, and cortisol, as well as the neurotransmitters dopamine and serotonin, also affect how organisms react to stress."* (Fight-or-Flight Response, *Wikipedia*,)

You need to listen to your body. For example, the emotion *anxiety* is telling you something stressful has been encountered. If left unresolved, it can become a constant disturbance in your daily life.

This is the point where you must be hungry for change instead of just thinking about it. It's also where you'll become educated about how stress affects your ability to make decisions.

For many of my clients, their emotional stress led to a physical problem, which is why I feel medication masks and numbs symptoms instead of addressing the cause. Once they get off the medication, the symptoms return very aggressively when their senses are reawakened.

Some individuals often get on the medication rollercoaster where they take them for a while, get off, then get back on. Working with a natural-minded health professional (naturopath) will help you to address the cause instead of the problem.

Mindfully monitoring your body is key to knowing what products or treatments to use. For instance, some of my clients won't do therapies that can help them get rid of old habits. So being aware of your body's signals will help you gain control over it and your mind.

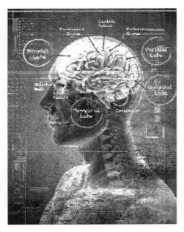

Whatever emotional or psychological trauma you're experiencing (i.e., stress, anxiety, depression, etc.), your hypothalamus, pituitary and hypothalamic-pituitary-adrenal axis (HPA) become activated, which causes a major shift in your body's basic functions and propel it into a state of stress. Think about a 911 dispatch center (your body). The dispatcher first takes all the information from the caller (hypothalamus), then relays it (pituitary) to the police or the fire department (adrenal) that organizes the information so that action can be taken.

The more your body is stimulated by fear, the more it becomes hardwired to the stress stimulus that causes a fight-or-flight response. If you don't get this under control, over time your body will lose the ability to have a high-functioning immune system, effectively reproduce cells, maintain healthy digestion, and manage other daily functions, all of which create havoc within your body.

Without parasympathetic activity (which is how the body rebuilds itself and relaxes), you'll struggle with longevity and vitality.

Some extreme situations can also cause a parasympathetic issue. But that's a different issue that can be measured by many kinds of biofeedback (biofeedback as Heart Variability, SDNN, and other forms; not the recent types of quantum biofeedback).

## How Do You Know if You're Dealing With Sympathetic Lock or Fight-or-Flight Reactions?

Let me quickly explain the difference between *parasympathetic* and *sympathetic* nervous systems. Simply stated, the parasympathetic slows things like your heart rate down in your body. Whereas the sympathetic accelerates them by releasing adrenaline into your system.

For example, if you're idling at a stop light, and are frustrated because the traffic isn't moving, your body doesn't know why you're upset. It goes into a "fight" mode as though it was preparing for battle. Parasympathetic slows your body down so you can handle the situation sensibly and without stress.

The following lists are red flags to let you know when you're dealing with certain fears and anxieties that keep you frozen, or make you want to run for the hills. They're also signs that the adrenals are beginning to become weaker:

You can't tolerate...

- repetitive sounds or loud noise
- physical touch
- decreased sexual activity or drive
- crowds
- conflict

You often feel...

- easily startled
- jumpy or on edge
- easily angered
- stressed
- irritated
- frustrated

You might not relate to a few or all of the above. But you might identify with ones that resonate with experiences you've had.

As time goes on, it will be imperative to clear any negative thoughts, smells, visions, images, etc., related to the experience. Then once your body is at rest, it can become more relaxed and function much better. You'll still remember the situation, but your emotions will no longer be strongly tied to it.

Sometimes with chronic stress your endocrine system needs to be supported with supplements, essential oils, and homeopathic treatments to help you deal with the lack of energy, or a feeling that your healing is progressing too slow.

(This is especially true for veterans coming back from war. Since their bodies are in terrible disarray, their physical and energetic fields need to be supported to bring about change and ultimate relief.)

Holistic treatments, that often include essential oils, can be made by an individual trained in the field of homeopathy. (There are many great books or websites on homeopathy, but that's beyond the scope of this book. I can also create them for you, so contact WPHC for more information.)

Emotions associated with trauma live right underneath the surface of your thoughts. So you shouldn't push them into the recesses of your subconscious where they can trigger emotions like fear or rage. This might help you stay numb, but it doesn't teach your body how to self-regulate. Instead, they need to be faced and dealt with so they don't keep controlling your life.

Emotions can be a great way to gain insight into how you're doing if you don't want to stay numb. Because a numb state of being doesn't sense joy, it tries to avoid the deep states of anger or depression.

## Understanding the Fight-or-Flight Response

The kind of trauma I'm discussing isn't tangible, like losing an arm or a leg (which of course causes its own kind of trauma). But *perceived* trauma that lingers in the recesses of your subconscious.

At this point you might thinking that you don't have a big "T" trauma in your life. However, I'm not only talking about big traumas, but little "t" traumas as well. For example, a child not being picked first for kickball can create the feeling of *why don't they like me?* Or an adult not being given a promotion can create the same feelings of self-doubt.

If not corrected and viewed differently, over time those thoughts can turn into *I never win*, and *people don't like me.*

Individuals with unresolved trauma often see daily events from a negative perspective, as the initial event overloaded the brain's trauma networks (i.e., the hippocampus and other parts of the brain). Things can become much bigger than they need to be.

- *That car cut in front of me. Now I'll be late to work!* (might cause road rage)

- *I can't believe Susie came down with a cold. Now I have to miss my special yoga session again!* (might cause embarrassment, a sleepless night, and possibly also catching a cold due to stress)

So it's good to know that trauma can affect your brain's anatomy, and that it's not something you imagine.

Being over-aroused and stimulated can cause you to see almost everything from a negative perspective, which can put you into a sympathetic lock (the flight-or-flight response). People who remain in a deep state beyond fight-or-flight stay "frozen" (this isn't my term, but one researchers are exploring). Their body is an in increased state of awareness, and a heightened state of alert.

For example, if you've ever had someone actually break into your house, just thinking back on the experience could make you relive the feeling of being paralyzed and not knowing what to do. This will cause your body to go into *sympathetic lock*, and create 14,000 biochemical and molecular responses within your body.

*"An avalanche of physiological changes begins, including increased muscle tension, breathing, brain wave frequency, blood pressure and heart rate, and decreased skin temperature."* (Demos, *Getting Started With Neurofeedback*, 2005)

Fight-or-flight isn't often essential for people constantly dealing with financial, unresolved emotional issues, messy homes, stress at work, fussy kids, negative self-talk, computer problems, etc. (though you might feel like packing your bags and running away from home when you become overwhelmed).

However, an individual with PTSD will go straight into the defense or fight-or-flight mode. At that point, there are numerous triggers that appear to be a serious threat (*appear* being important to remember, as most often the threat is only *perceived* as real).

Everyday events can seem to be much bigger than in reality (a learned response to environmental activities for those dealing with trauma). For example, in a mind experiencing trauma, a tiny spider might look like a gigantic tarantula. Hence, the perception that there's a need to go into action and kill it, jump on a chair, or run from the room.

Although the person's body might not recognize a non-life-threatening emotional response, it can cause the same physiological response as a soldier going into battle, or a serious car accident where fight-or-flight is necessary to avoid being blown up.

Oftentimes when the body goes into a false sense of fight-or-flight, as opposed to a real occurrence when it needs resources to survive, it lacks sufficient logic to get through the event. The rebuilding process to regaining your health can become compromised if you stay locked in fear, and you don't know which way to turn.

Actions and responses are caused from perceptions and emotions typically based on an individual's lifestyle and subjective viewpoints. For example, when stuck in traffic your mind thinks about financial stress, or an argument with your spouse, instead of focusing on what's in front of you.

## Listening to Your Body's Signals

Following is an excerpt from the study, "A Meta-Analysis of Heart Rate Variability as a Psychophysiological Indicator of Posttraumatic Stress Disorder" (Nagpal et al):

*Posttraumatic stress disorder (PTSD) syndrome is accompanied by the changes in autonomic nervous system, and heart rate variability (HRV) parameters assess the balance of sympathetic and parasympathetic influences on heart rate. HRV is a promising psychophysiological indicator of PTSD. The aim of this meta-analysis is to provide a quantitative account of the literature findings on PTSD and co-occurring HRV parameters. We first examined the effect size of PTSD on HRV in available published studies, and we then examined the effects of PTSD treatments on various HRV parameters.*

This study demonstrates that the power of HRV can have an impact on, and is exceptional for, psychophysicological indicators and treatment.

So how can your body and/or mind know what to do if you're not aware enough to take charge of the situation?

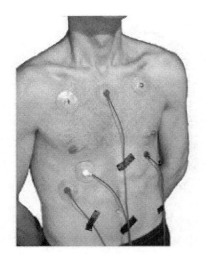

To monitor your fight-or-flight responses, you'll first observe your resting heart rate – a great tool to understand what your body is trying to tell you – which should be below 80 beats per minute (bpm).

You can also monitor skin temperature which should be around 88 to 92 degrees Fahrenheit. This is an indicator of good parasympathetic activity.

I often see traumatized individuals with resting heart rates of 105 bpm with a skin temperature of 78, and some as high as 130 bpm with a low skin temperature around 68. As fight-or-flight begins to set in (but not while in a state of rage), a person's heart rate will often be around 80 to 100 bpm.

Determining your pulse rate can be done several ways. The best location is a soft "cushion" on your neck directly below your eyes under the jawline where you'll feel your heart beating. Using a clock with a second hand, stopwatch, or a cell phone app, you can measure it in units of 15, 20, 30 seconds, etc. (I often use 15 seconds, then multiple it times 4.)

For example, if you use 15 seconds, when the clock hits 15 you stop counting. If you get 20 beats in that amount of time, multiple it times 4 which would equal 80 beats per minute (20x4=80 bpm).

(Skin conductance measurement devices can be purchased from websites, and cost around twenty-five dollars.)

*NOTE: If you're on any prescription or over-the-counter medication, your pulse numbers might be very different, and won't be an accurate reflection of what your body is trying to tell you. If you have others issues, and feel your results are worrisome, discuss your concerns with your healthcare provider immediately.*

What was your pulse number? _____

What was your skin temperature? _____

On a scale of 9 to 10, how would you rate your stress level (10 being the most stressed you've ever been, and 0 not stressed at all)?:

_____

Do you feel calm or frustrated? _____ Yes _____ No

If yes, explain what you're feeling, and what caused those feelings.

_____
_____
_____

If your pulse rate was over 80, and your skin temperature below 80, do you feel on edge, anxious or keyed up? _____ Yes _____ No

If yes, can you identify any emotions associated with that state?

_____
_____
_____

# Exercise:
## Fight-or-Flight and Essential Oils

*NOTE: If you have a lung condition or other conditions that could cause this to be difficult, then please check with your physician before you begin doing any of these activities as they are only intended to help you to relax.*

Put several drops of lavender, lemon, cedarwood, palo santo, and frankincense essential oils into the well of your hand, say a quick prayer over them, and stir them on your hand clockwise. Then apply the oils to the base of the back of your neck.

Apply peppermint and rosemary oil on top of your head. And vetiver and ylang ylang from your belly button up to your nose.

Then do the same on your back from your belt line up your spine to the top of your head. (If you have no one to help, you can find instructions on the Internet, or just do the best you can. There are long dowel tools with end applicators that might help.)

Place several drops of orange, fennel, marjoram, cypress and peppermint in the well of your hand, stir clockwise with your fingertip, then rub the oil on your entire stomach area.

Then place several drops of geranium oil in the same hand, stir clockwise, and apply to the skin over your heart.

Then either with a stopwatch or watching a clock, count how many times you breathe during one (1) minute.

You might have tried breathing exercises in the past, and felt like they did nothing for you. However, if you practice them as instructed in this workbook, you'll feel a bit light-headed or dizzy if you're a shallow breather (that's actually a good thing as it shows oxygen is getting into your bloodstream). If you aren't, you might not feel much.

People experiencing trauma might find they breathe 25 to 30 times per minute, which is how a shallow breather experiencing stress will breathe. This often creates a high pulse rate, and an unawareness of how stressed and tense they are.

Most people don't compare their stress levels with others as this type of conversation can be difficult or awkward. They might have a high stress threshold level, but don't know how to determine it.

While reading this book you might wonder where your stress level is at, but don't have a clue as to what it is.

The use of biofeedback to determine stress levels would be unlikely to come up in a routine conversation. The science of measuring tension and other phenomena in your body can teach you how stressed and tense you are, which is called "conditioning" or training your body to be more efficient and healthy.

A simple way to test stress is to check your pulse by placing two fingertips on the inside of your wrist below your thumb where the artery is (don't use your thumb because it has its own pulse).

Count your heartbeats for 30 seconds, then double that amount to get the number of beats per minute. If you're feeling frustrated, your heart rate can rise very fast to 100. If it's over 100 bpm, you're experiencing way too much stress and/or a medical issue. You'll go into fight-or-flight mode, and your body will be put on "autopilot," so to speak.

However, if you're taking medication and your bpm is around 60, that's great. But you might not really know how you're doing as the medication can lower your pulse rate. So if you're un-medicated, you want your resting heart rate to be 60 to 80 bpms.

A proper resting heart rate creates a good level of heart coherence that creates a stronger baroreflex (a term used to describe balance). The current theory is your heart is the strongest electrical generator of your body.

Your heart's electrical activity can be measured upwards of eight feet. When your heart and brain become in sync, you'll begin to feel relaxed. When your brain and heart are out of sync, you'll experience more stress and tension. You might feel cold, your heart might beat faster, and you might experience more muscle tension, which can cause your body to be further out of balance (homeostasis).

## Breathing the Right Way to Help You Relax

You might not know there's a right and wrong way to breathe. You need to learn the *right* way to breathe, especially when incorporating essential oils into your healing regimen.

There are numerous factors that go into the math and science of breathing. But this type of breathing will increase the resonance in your breathing patterns and help you to relax more.

Combining visualization with essential oils, the following exercise will activate the parasympathetic portion of your brain that controls your well-being and vitality if you can remain in this state. (I've used this method to measure vibrational increases in my clients, and the results are awesome!)

As you breathe and relax, your skin temperature will rise (you can use a simple alcohol thermometer to test it, or purchase a digital meter online). This is due to sympathetic lock in that the body re-routes blood to stay more centralized in your body. Then as you relax, blood circulates better throughout your entire body.

*NOTE: If you have no medical restrictions, it's okay to do this exercise. However, if you've taken any prescription or over-the-counter medication, your results might not be accurate.*

Before you do this exercise, check your blood pressure and your pulse. I've seen people lower both. In some cases, so much so that I couldn't believe it.

BP: _____/ _____
Pulse:_____

- First, breathe chamomile or any relaxing oil of your choice. Count to 6 as you inhale. While inhaling, your stomach and chest should move together.

- Exhale while counting to 8, and pushing on your stomach with both hands. (If you can talk, air is still in your lungs.) Exhaling properly is important because it supports your parasympathetic nervous system, and creates heart rate coherence.

- Repeat once.

- Now cup your hands over your nose, and continue to breathe in the oil vapors at 8 to 10 breaths per minute rate to activate the parasympathetic portion of your central nervous system. Do this for several minutes.

- Monitor your pulse rate again, and write down any changes:

Pulse rate before _____
Pulse rate after _____
Skin temperature before: _____
Skin temperature after (remember sometimes skin temp will rise slowly): _____

Stress level before this exercise on a scale of 0 to 10 (10 being the most stressed, 0 not stressed at all): _____

Stress level after this exercise on a scale of 0 to 10: _____

What kinds of emotions were you experiencing before this exercise?

_____

_____

_____

_____

What kinds of emotions are you feeling after this exercise?

_____

_____

_____

_____

Doing this exercise often will keep you grounded and relaxed during the day. (You can use this technique along with other techniques in the next chapter to help you sleep better.)

Now that you've learned that essential oils can help you breathe better, in the next chapter you'll learn how they help you sleep better.

# Essential Oils
# Can Help You Sleep Better

Do your physical or emotional problems or traumas prevent you from getting a good night's sleep? Do you toss and turn, then get out of bed to watch a late night movie, or work at your laptop because you can't sleep?

Do you wake up in the morning feeling tired and unrested?

During the day your body has to defend itself against bacteria, viruses, toxins, and other foreign invaders. It's also busy digesting food, eliminating waste, repairing cells, and numerous other functions to keep your body's systems working properly.

Because your body is designed to rejuvenate while it rests, a good night's sleep is one of the most essential elements to a quality existence. Rebuilding all of its cells every two years require a great deal of energy, so not sleeping well will decrease your body's ability to be healthy.

## It's Imperative to Get a Good Night's Rest!

Instant gratification is prevalent in today's busy world, so it can be difficult to see the daily improvements that will get you to where you want to be. Things you want to pay attention to that indicate you're beginning to heal are waking up less, feeling more rested when you wake up, and taking less time to go to bed.

Stress, trauma, or physical issues can prevent you from getting the rest your body deserves. Unfortunately, people don't try to deal with their problems so they can have a restful night's sleep.

Over the years I've met many people who are always on the go and barely take time to eat and get enough rest. I don't mean people who live a busy but well-balanced life. I mean people who always need to be physically moving, often because their mind races with thoughts they're trying to keep up with.

*Being constantly busy doesn't always mean being productive.*

Not finding moments to be still can cause them to be less dependent on sleep, which can be very destructive to their entire body.

Also, consuming energy drinks or stimulating food before going to bed disrupts natural sleep patterns and heightens brain frequency. If you have a hard time going to sleep, stop drinking or eating anything that could stimulate your body and mind at least six hours before going to bed.

## Using an Essential Oil Diffuser at Night

Using essential oils works for many other issues other than PTSD. For instance, like Jason's subconscious memories of gunfire and explosions, emotional responses can be triggered by smells, loud sounds, and many other things within your environment.

While searching for an essential oil that would help his emotional issues, he found a sweet citrus oil blend that exceeded his expectations. Applying it every night to his temples, the middle of his forehead, around his navel and on his big toes, he slept better than he had in a long time.

After a few weeks, Jason's dreams contained peaceful memories of childhood and family events. This was a significant sign that he was on the road to wellness as he'd blocked out the years prior to being eight years old.

I once worked with a veteran who loved the smell of ruta oil (aka: rue, or herb-of-grace). Using it in a diffuser, he reported sleeping well throughout the night. Though I personally don't find the smell very pleasant, or would recommend it for any other purpose, it possesses many relaxing properties. (Remember, personal preference plays a big part in diffusing oils. You can refer back to the section where I discuss how to change an oil's smell to something you enjoy.)

Diffusing relaxing oils at night such as lavender, lemon, frankincense, helichrysum, neroli, vetiver, ylang ylang, and cedarwood can help you slip into a comfortable, deep sleep.

Diffusing an oil 30 to 60 minutes before going to bed allows the oil's molecules to saturate the room.

Once you snuggle into bed, use the oil in conjunction with a deep breathing exercise to help you drift off to sleep. You'll awaken refreshed, alert, and ready for whatever the next day brings!

## The Science of Sleep

Scientists have found that emotional trauma affects brain. With trauma, there might be an increase in slow brain waves (sadness), and very fast brain waves (stress). When the brain goes too fast, and the circadian rhythms are out of balance, it will be difficult to have a clear mind in order to relax and fall asleep.

For example, someone who's sad or depressed might experience a decrease in their body's ability to reset and rejuvenate. So a good night's sleep helps the body to rejuvenate and recharge your "batteries."

### The Five Stages of Sleep

There are five sleep cycles your body needs to go through to enter a state of rejuvenation, which includes the first four stages of non-REM (rapid eye movement) sleep and one of REM sleep.

***Non-REM Stages*** (from Frank Lawlis's book, *The PTSD Breakthrough*)

Stage 1 is the transition period between being awake and fully asleep. Anxiety and insomnia can lengthen this period, and make it difficult to transition to deeper states of sleep.

Individuals with intense insomnia might never make it past this point, which can tax the body's restoration process. This stage occurs for 2 to 5% of the normal night sleep.

Stage 2 is characterized as the beginning of deep sleep where your heart rate slows and your body temperature can drop. This stage also can have different effects on the healing process. Stage two often accounts for about 45 to 60% of a normal night's sleep.

Stages 3 and 4 are considered the final two, deeper periods of sleep. During these non-REM stages, your body repairs itself by rebuilding tissue, bone and muscle, and strengthening the immune system. During these stages, the brain enters a deep delta frequency.

Lawlis points out that: "Contrary to popular belief, it is this delta sleep that is the 'deepest' stage of sleep (not REM), and is what a sleep-deprived person's brain craves the most. In adults it can last from 15 to 30 minutes. In children it can occupy up to 40% of all sleep time..." (which is why it's difficult to wake children during most of the night).

## Achieving REM

"After REM sleep, the body usually returns to stage 2 sleep. You can have many cycles through sleep." (Lawlis)

Stage 5 rapid eye movement (REM) sleep typically happens 90 minutes after you fall asleep. The first round typically lasts 10 minutes. Each of your later REM stages gets longer, and the final one may last up to an hour.

When your heart rate and breathing quickens, and your eyes move under your eyelids (ergo, the rapid eye movement), you might experience vivid dreams.

If you feel tired after you awaken, review the five stages of sleep. Most people who can't slow down their brain won't reach the delta stages to reach deep sleep.

For example, for clients dealing with trauma, their brain maps reveal that they are never fully awake or asleep. So during the day, their brain slows and at night it goes too fast (referred to as delta/theta issues). Over time, issues with their circadian rhythms and pineal gland make it more difficult to break difficult sleep patterns.

Begin being consistently diffusing an oil every night. Give it several months because you'll need time to stop the pattern. Your body will want to sleep, so this will help relax it and achieve balance.

A good technique to help with rebalancing your circadian rhythms is to take frankincense oil outside. During this exercise *don't look at the sun directly*, but off to the side.

- Put a drop of oil on your fingertip, then place it on the center of your forehead.

- With your eyes open, look up at the sun (near it, only as close as comfortable) for 5 minutes.

- Then close your eyes for 5 minutes while doing the breathing exercise.

- Do this exercise for 3 sets which would be a total of 30 minutes. If you don't have that amount of time, do it for at least one cycle of ten minutes. I've had people break it into 3 minutes with their eyes open and 3 minutes with their eyes closed for two cycles (12 minutes total).

# Exercise:
## Analyzing Your Sleep Patterns

It's always good to monitor and record how things are changing as you're making modifications to your lifestyle. So take a few moments to document what it was like before you start (or have already begun) using essential oils:

Do you have a hard time going to sleep? _____ Yes _____ No

If yes, write down why (i.e., your thoughts don't stop, you eat before you go to bed, you're worried about your job and/or family, etc.)?

_____

_____

_____

When you wake up, do you feel well-rested? _____ Yes _____ No

Do you need caffeine (coffee, tea, Red Bull, etc.) to get you going in the morning? _____ Yes _____ No

If yes, how much do you drink? _____

Do you drink alcohol to slow down in the evening in order to help yourself go to sleep? _____ Yes _____ No

If yes, how often do you do this (every night, whenever needed, etc.)?

_____

How much do you consume? _____

How long does it normally take to fall asleep? _____

How many times do you normally wake up during the night?

_____

Do you often wake up during the night seemingly for no reason? _____ Yes _____ No

Have you experienced night terrors and bad dreams? _____ Yes _____ No

If yes, how often? _____

Do you sleep in a room with an LCD television on? (asking because the displaced color blue can cause neurochemical issues)
_____ Yes _____ No

Do you have restless leg syndrome (RLS)? _____ Yes _____ No

Do you have hot flashes during the night? _____ Yes _____ No

If so how often do they happen? _____

Do you feel your time awake and your sleep cycles are in sync with the sun (this is important for the production of melatonin)?
_____ Yes _____ No

If no, were they while growing up (this shows things changed when you became an adult with responsibilities and worries)?
_____ Yes _____ No

Because change might occur slowly over time, you might not feel you've made much progress. But being able to fall asleep in 45 minutes instead of 90 minutes is a great sign of improvement.

Write down your sleep patterns to see if you're making any improvement in following the sun's rhythms:

_____
_____
_____
_____

Try using your diffuser with your favorite oil along with this exercise for the next 45 nights to see how you are doing.

# The Power of Attraction

While observing married couples at my office, I've often wondered how they met and made their marriage work. Did they attract a person of a similar vibration, while repelling others whose vibrations didn't resonate with theirs?

You sense so much unconsciously, that pulling to consciousness can change everything about you, and what and who you attract.

## Belief *Can* Change Your Energy

One year I was dealing with many different, and sometimes difficult issues. But everything changed when I used all the tools in my arsenal. For example, a shipping issue was causing multiple complications. Combining an essential oil with an affirmation and prayer shifted my mindset to believing the issue would stop. And it did!

According to the Law of Cause and Effect, you attract what you're in vibration with. If you believe you're not worthy of receiving, that's exactly what you'll attract. Therefore, you hold the key to the kinds of things you say, and the thoughts you have, to manifest whatever you desire.

People thrive in, or are just trying to survive in, the spiritual realm. By healing your issues, and learning to be in control of your emotions, you'll be restored to your correct frequency. You'll then become a beacon of light to help guide others toward their healing.

## Exercise:
## Attract the Right People and Situations

What negative and positive things, events and people have you attracted throughout your life?

_____

_____

_____

_____

_____

_____

What do you want to change about the negativity you're attracting? It could be people, events, situations, your job, your friendships or marriage, etc.

_____

_____

_____

_____

_____

From that list, choose the one that feels like the most difficult to cope with.

_____

_____

What do you think could be the first step toward turning this negative attraction into a positive one?

_____

_____

_____

_____

While working on your issues you can constantly return to this exercise (in fact, I highly suggest it). I work on my own personal issues all the time. For instance, as I sense an energy I want to change, I first pray about it. Then I speak to it, and use an oil plus an affirmation to release it.

One time when I had severe back pain, I could have spent a lot of money on numerous visits to traditional doctors, only to have them prescribe expensive medications that didn't work.

But when I felt the Lord telling me to listen to my body, I "heard" the pain was occurring due to an emotional imbalance. Once I began working on regaining emotional balance, the pain shifted and left.

By now you should realizing the benefits Jason, I and many others have received from essential oils and the treatments I'm discussing can happen to you as well!

# Affirmations, Meditation and Essential Oils to Clear Trauma

Have you ever been driving home, and later you don't remember the act of driving or how long it took you to get home? Something nagging you in your unconscious mind was probably prevented you from focusing on your environment.

Or do you know someone, including yourself, who's tried everything possible to get better? They've gone from doctor to doctor while spending a great deal of money, only to find that nothing works.

The Internet allows access to many alternative methods of healing the mind, body and spirit. There are many ways to clear whatever is causing your trauma so you can begin the healing process.

## Affirmations

From Dr. Carmen Hara's article on "35 Affirmations That Will Change Your Life":

*"Affirmations are proven methods of self-improvement because of their ability to rewire our brains. Much like exercise, they raise the level of feel-good hormones and push our brains to form new clusters of 'positive thought' neurons. In the sequence of thought-speech-action, affirmations play an integral role by breaking patterns of negative thoughts, negative speech, and, in turn, negative actions."*

The art of the spoken word is critical in crafting our futures. As a teacher of spirituality, it's my firm belief that the Universe is influenced word by word. If you dictate your wishes to it, it will respond.

When you utter sounds, you emit a sound wave into the Universe. The sound pierces the air and becomes a real object that exists in the world intangibly and invisibly.

No words are empty words, as every syllable we speak engages energy towards or against us. For instance, if you constantly say 'I can't,' the energy of your words will repel the universal force against you. But if you say 'I can!' the Universe will endow you with the abilities to do just that.

Another great resource is Dr. Corinne Allen's book, *Light Beyond Trauma*, where she discusses a script she created to remove trauma blocks with essential oils. (Her DVD set is available for sale; plus there's a mini-trailer on her website where she discusses her brain program.)

*"It is well-documented that proper types of stimulation will cause the brain to grow more neural connections. It is documented that powerful ways to stimulate new brain connections are: light color, sound music movement nutrition touch oxygen."*

# CASE STUDY ONE:
## Thinking Outside the Box

Typically, people who come to see me have both physical and emotional issues. Individuals who've been living with pain for a long period of time, or haven't found relief through traditional medicine, often feel their pain is untreatable.

However, I've educated many people on how I've achieved good results with HRV biofeedback, tapping, tuning forks, frequency, voltage and essential oils to help support medical intervention.

For example, one day a man named Brett (who'd been referred by his friend to come in to WPHC for an assessment) came to my office as he'd been experiencing chronic life-altering, low-grade headaches. Though they weren't painful cluster migraines, they were preventing him from having a quality life.

When asked what he'd done in the past to get rid of them, he said, "Everything."

His doctor had originally prescribed a very high pain relief medication over a period of six months, which Brett continued to use for several years. Initially it helped alleviate his headaches.

But during a routine checkup, they realized it was possibly causing problems. They switched him to a different medication, which didn't work as well as the first one.

Relying solely on the medication might have eased his medical symptoms. But it didn't empower him to take charge of his wellness. So I explored Brett's pain levels, and how his central nervous system (CNS) was handling the stress.

There are natural central alpha agonists (CAAs) that can help reduce sympathetic nervous system (SNS) responses, such as...

- celery and celery seed oil
- coenzyme Q10 (CoQ10)
- fiber
- gamma-linolenic acid (GLA) -- an Omega-6 fatty acid
- garlic
- taurine
- vitamins K, B-6 and C
- zinc

I instructed Brett on how to use an HRV diaphragm breathing method to support his circulation and decrease overstimulation. Preventing his CNS from becoming overstimulated would allow his body to relax more, and have a better parasympathetic response. He was amazed at how this method helped decrease his blood pressure and balance his skin temperature.

Using essential oils and affirmations between sessions accelerated his belief and healing response. Over time, Brett became more balanced during our sessions, and he wasn't dealing with as much pain.

An affirmation we used together (both saying "I"): *I choose to release all layers of pain in all parts of my being that no longer serve me.*

Brett used 3 drops each of clove, frankincense, helicrysum, rosemary, lemon and marjoram on his feet and back 4 to 8 times every day. At first he didn't like the smell, so he used affirmations to remove the trauma associated with the negative smell.

Since exercising is hands down one of the best things a person can have in their wellness protocol, using the oils and affirmations increased Brett's stamina. Based on what his doctor told him he could do, he'd start slowly, then would stop if the pain became too much.

Although it wasn't a quick fix, Brett stayed with the program. After about a month-and-a-half, he reported that people were commenting on a noticeable shift in his personality and moods.

Prior to coming to WPHC, Brett was disconnected from himself and his environment. During our sessions, he opened up about the pain in his heart because he'd realized that people didn't know the real him, and he didn't know who the people in his life really were. (This was part of the stress and distancing I noticed in his earlier sessions. But I left it alone as I knew it would surface when the time was right.)

Although he was now feeling happier, he admitted to having stayed busy so he wouldn't have to face the loneliness and isolation. After three months of working hard to reconnect to himself, he went back to his doctor and asked to be taken off his medication.

## Facing Then Releasing Negative Emotions

In addition to Dr. Allen's *The Script* (referenced below), I'd like to suggest reading *Releasing Emotional Patterns With Essential Oils* by Dr. Carolyn Mein as it lists emotions, the other side of emotions, and the way out of the emotions. Plus the kinds of oil to use (Dr. Mein includes a chart of the points where you'll place the oil).

A few of the primary emotions Dr. Mein discusses that need to be released to clear trauma are:

- abandonment
- abuse
- anger
- anxiety
- blame
- criticism
- control
- deception
- denial
- fear
- guilt
- jealousy
- pain
- rage
- rejection
- resentment
- shame

*"Believe in yourself! Have faith in your abilities!*
*Without a humble but reasonable confidence in your own powers, you*
*cannot be successful or happy."*
~Norman Vincent Peale

Louise Hay's book, *Heal Your Body: The Mental Causes for Physical Illness and the Metaphysical Way to Overcome Them*, provides terrific affirmations to overcome your issues.

For instance, under *anxiety* she writes, "Not trusting the flow and process of life." And the following affirmations: "I love and approve myself. I trust the process of life. I am safe."

Studies on how much birth trauma affects a person's life are on the rise. Some professionals believe people's personalities are formed during fetal development. Originating in the ectoderm, the neural plate is later formed in the brain, which is how a fetus receives its emotions before coming into the world.

Simply put, the fetus receives its emotions from their mother's hormones. For example, an imbalance in cortisol can create a host of emotions. Experiencing stress during a woman's pregnancy can create low self-worth, insecurity, and other emotional issues that can manifest later in life.

Following is an affirmation from Dr. Corinne Allen's trauma release script. Frankincense is one of the best oils to use, unless you have Idaho blue spruce available to you which would be preferable. This affirmation is repeated three times:

*I choose to release the trauma behind the trapped emotion of _____ that no longer serves me in a positive and productive way.*

For example, "I choose to release the trauma behind the trapped emotion of rage that no longer serves me in a positive and productive way."

Following is a client case study where affirmations, essential oils and brain mapping (neuroscience) were utilized help this individual lose childhood trauma-induced weight.

## CASE STUDY TWO:
## Losing Weight in the Mind, Body and Spirit

"Struggling with mood issues for years, I had done a lot of work with my doctor and a therapist. Feeling stuck, I'd been reading a few different things online. Searching for someone local to go to, I found Watson Psychological Health Center [WPHC in Amarillo].

When I came to Ryan for help with my depression – plus childhood memories I hadn't been able to talk about with anyone – he went over all the different types of therapies we could try. We first decided to do a brain map, then neurofeedback where I began to feel more relaxed and calm.

As I began to feel better, we moved into Eye Movement Desensitization and Reprocessing (EMDR), and techniques for emotional release.

To begin this process he created affirmations, and chose specific essential oils to enhance them. Ryan then used a gas discharge visualization camera [the Biowell image system mentioned earlier] to determine which emotions were affecting me.

I've always had weight issues. But none of the doctors knew why, and nothing I did seemed to help. Using the affirmations and the essential oils together, I felt more comfortable talking about my childhood in order to understand what might have created them early in life.

After doing the affirmations and oils for several weeks, we did an incredible emotional release session. At first I didn't think it would help because I felt overwhelmed by sensations I hadn't felt in a long time. I didn't know what to do with everything that was surfacing. Begin calm and patient, Ryan walked me through everything.

The next day I felt great! The heaviness I was so use to, and never realized I was feeling, was much less. So much so that I noticed it without really thinking about it.

Then I began working on EMDR to face my childhood memories. I diffused the oils every night and began working on my trauma triggers inventory.

I actually found EMDR to be easy and freeing. I learned that due to my childhood issues, I didn't want to be or feel pretty. I also learned that I had done this on purpose to protect myself without noticing I was doing it.

Over time I found it was much easier to eat the way I wanted, and I began to lose weight. Now I really enjoy being around people, and I'm no longer sensitive to every little thing. Plus, I find it's easier to think more positive thoughts and see myself more positively.

To this day I continue to use my affirmations and oils. I look and feel so much better. I wish I would have done this years ago!" ~Sarah from Texas

# Using Biowell Technology to Reveal Emotional Trauma

Gas Discharge Visualization technology is a great way to understand the body's gasses and electrical flow.

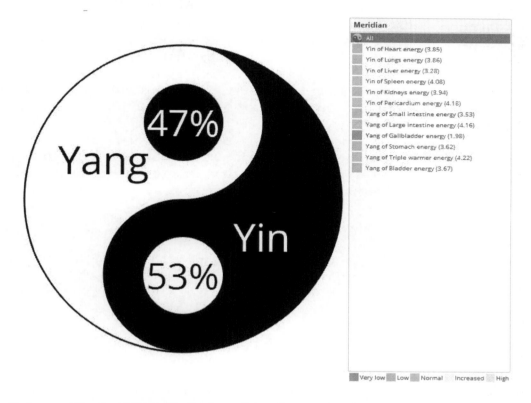

Taken with the Biowell device, this shows the image of the energy tab along with the energy levels of the different meridians of the body. Green is normal, and only a few are normal during the first recording.

This individual, who was going through a divorce, had never gone through counseling or other therapy. They'd never done this or any other kind of tests, so their belief and faith in its value was low. But because they wanted to do whatever would be best for their healing, at first I chose to focus on any birth and generational trauma they might have had (I discuss more on this in the section "From the Day You Were Born" in the chapter *Eliminating Negative Thoughts and Self-Talk*).

Since no one has control over these types of traumas as they're acquired genetically, I've found that emotional, birth, and heart traumas often need to be worked on separately.

They're hard to measure if you don't know what you're dealing with. But in my client's case, it was imperative to be done, which is why I used the Biowell device to measure theirs.

It was interesting that their parents' relationship was extremely strained during their mother's pregnancy. The father was physically abusive to his wife. The more I and my client uncovered their traumas, the clearer it became that anxiety was a huge issue for his mother. She didn't feel safe due to the husband's abuse, so her anxiety and panic about most things carried over to her baby in utero.

Because this individual's life began very turbulently, they also didn't feel safe. So it's easy to see that anxiety became natural reaction for them as they grew up.

After our discussions, a second Biowell test showed their balance was nearly perfect at 50/50 split. Talk about a drastic change once their problems were determined!

## Meditation

Meditation has been known to have profound effects on a person's alpha state brain waves (presented relaxed state of being) while taking an EEG (a test that measures and records electrical activity in the brain).

To get into the state of stillness and presence (alpha) requires a person to be still, and enter a place of oneness with all of their life's experiences. Based on my observations, oils that help achieve this state are frankincense, lemon, lavender and Idaho blue spruce (this is only based on my observations). They can be used during prayer, meditation or other such activities.

Meditating allows you to calm down instead of slowing down. Plus, it can move you into a more positive state of being or vibration so you can be in a tranquil alpha state of mind.

I usually begin with trying to introduce the "state of nothingness," as I and others call it. This is where you control your brain by not thinking about anything at all, which takes mental control and focus.

You can begin a number of different ways, such as meditating on anything you like (health, career, relationships, finances, etc.). If you struggle to find something to meditate on, you might have not completed the earlier exercise to determine the issue(s) you're having.

If you did complete that exercise, review the list and choose an item to include in the meditation below.

The following is from Karol Truman's book, *Feelings Buried Alive Never Die* – just one example of any kind of meditation you can use (they're all over the Internet; just choose which one feels right for you). She also goes into great detail about buried emotions, which will be beneficial while determining which one(s) you're trying to face and deal with:

*"Spirit/Super-Conscious, please locate the origin of my feeling(s) thought(s) of _____ [insert whatever you're dealing with]. Take each and every level, layer, area, and aspect of my Be-ing to this origin. Then analyze and resolve it perfectly with God's truth."*

Following is an example of a meditation to help ease anger:

*"Spirit/Super-Conscious, please locate the origin of my feeling(s) thought(s) of rage. Take each and every level, layer, area, and aspect of my Be-ing to this origin. Then analyze and resolve it perfectly with God's truth."*

During meditation, the above script will help build a bridge between your brain's two hemispheres in order for them to effectively communicate with each other.

It will also help remove any negative mindset (your paradigm mentioned earlier) remaining in your subconscious, and instill the positive paradigm you're working toward.

This will create a shift for emotions and feelings you have in your heart, and begin building a foundation on which to work.

# Exercise:
# Using Meditation to Remove Emotional and/or Spiritual Blocks

Using the correct meditation (the intention to which you give an issue) or affirmation to clear an emotion isn't a one-time fix, so you'll need to do this exercise on a daily basis.

I typically have clients do affirmations for 30 days while tracking what they felt before and afterwards. Oftentimes they might experience a calmer, more relaxed state almost immediately. While other times they might not notice anything at all.

It's not just about the feelings you experience. But also doing the work while keeping in mind the more affirmations you do, the better you'll feel. Memorizing the scripts will make it easier to say them any time during a day.

In addition to affirmations and meditation, you can use a frequency-containing device such as an essential oil, magnet, laser, or other devices to remove blocks preventing you from moving forward. (Magnets and lasers can be expensive, but the oils work just as well.)

Find a safe area where you can do this unclothed, as this can get a bit messy:

- First rub geranium oil on the base of your neck.

- Then rub Frankincense onto both wrist pulse points. Hold yours wrists together at those points while inhaling deeply while counting to five (holding them together in your lap, or on a tabletop, will keep them steady).

- Exhale while counting to five until a vibration is felt. Then firmly state, "I choose to release the heart blocks that are essential for this time to be cleared."

- Next you'll put 3 drops each of pine and peppermint into the well of your hand (meaning, cupped like you were going to put water into it). Then stir the oil clockwise 3 times.

  Using your fingertips, place the oil on the top of your head, then inhale and notice how you feel. Then cup your hands over your nose and breathe in the vapors 3 times. Pay attention to any subtle sense of peace and calmness about you (it will be subtle for some, while for others it will be much more noticeable). Opening your mind prepares you for the work that lies ahead.

- Place a few drops of basil, clary sage, cedarwood, helichrysum, lemon, lavender and marjoram into the palm of your hand. Stir clockwise to mix them together, then rub the oil on the skin over your heart.

  Then "paint" a steady line of oil on the front of your body from the belt line to the top of your head. Then from the top of your head down the other side of your body to just above the anus (you might need to dip your finger into the oil several times to create a steady stream).

As you do this repeat, say "I choose to release the trauma or negative emotion at the _____ (birth, emotional, or heart level you want to release) three times while rubbing the oil into your skin.

An example of an exercise I do with clients:

First. I have them put the oil on the front and back of their body. Then I have them say out loud, "I choose to release all levels of anger that no longer serve me" three times for each emotion or block being worked on. (In a roundabout way, a block or emotion is the same thing. In other words, an emotion blocked your healing at some point.)

Then move on to the next emotion. Remember, your issues need to be identified at all levels (birth, emotional, heart, and spiritual) in order to release negative emotions.

I use advanced techniques that require knowledge of many different systems and modalities. Since there are many books about emotions, pick the one(s) you resonate with (i.e., *Releasing Emotional Patterns with Essential Oils* by Dr. Mein is a great place to start). Don't be afraid to start, as trying is better than nothing, and eventually you'll become more creative. Allow your senses to guide this process as you can't mess anything up at this point.

- To hold on to the new vibration and where it's at in your body, place a few drops of lemon, peppermint, clary sage, sandalwood, myrrh, frankincense, lavender and palo santo into the palm of your hand. Stir them together, then place the oil on the pulse points of both wrists.

Place your wrists together while stating, "I choose to release all subconscious and conscious emotional blocks and traumas from my body that are no longer needed." Then, "I choose to receive love, peace and joy."

- Then put several drops of frankincense, balsam fir, copaiba, palo santo, lavender and orange into the well of your hand.

Apply a line of oil from the belt line to the top of the head, then from the top of the head to just above the anus (just like you did above), while stating, "I am ready to receive all that is intended for me as I am free from the emotional block now and forevermore. As I receive my healing, I am filled with love and joy."

Then, "I choose to accept and receive the positive transformation I am creating from this present moment to eternity."

Write down the physical and emotional sensations you've experienced:

_____

_____

_____

_____

_____

Remember, everyone's body has a different constitution, so it might take time to find what combinations of oils, affirmations and techniques work/don't work for you.

# Identifying and Managing Your Trauma and Associated Behavior and Emotional Patterns

U p to this point you've learned some basic, but powerful, tools and techniques that can help you shift your vibration. Now it's time to begin working on your mental paradigm (mindset).

To help illustrate the power of habits and cycles, and how you can get stuck in your thoughts, the emotional circle of cycles below is very beneficial (it's repeatedly used with numerous different emotions to get to the depth of the emotion):

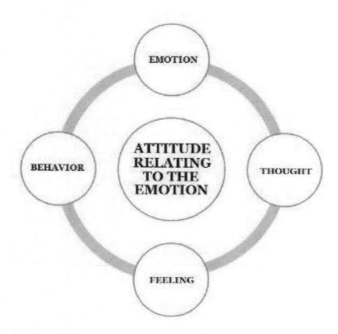

- Place the attitude relating to the emotion in the center circle.
- Place the emotion in the top circle.
- Place your thought about the emotion in the right-hand circle.
- Place your feeling about the emotion in the bottom circle.
- Place your behavior in the left-hand circle. Then head back up to the emotion circle.

Attitudes and beliefs are deeper than emotions. An attitude consists of numerous emotions. Attitudes combined with experiences create beliefs. You can have numerous cycles for many different attitudes and beliefs.

Using the example of anger for brain anatomy and physiology, there are many different types of anger (i.e., irritable aggression, defensive aggression, fear-induced aggression) and rage (I'm discussing these in terms of managing the primary emotion of fear).

The areas of the brain that are involved are:

- the thalamus (relay center for sensory information)
- the amygdala (the medial amygdala, specifically emotional stimulation from perceived sensory awareness)
- the hypothalamus (medial hypothalamus – controls autonomic function from sensory information).

Looking at these from an individual's perspective will determine how these areas of the brain are or are not activated. For instance, the sense of smell (oftentimes the aroma of an essential oil) can move the body out of sympathetic lock, thus allowing the person to be more relaxed and calm.

Changing your belief can rewire the neurons in your brain, which ultimately can change your behavior, thoughts, and ultimately your life.

## Freeing Yourself from Negative Self-Talk and Doubts

*"Those who guard their mouths and their tongues*
*keep themselves from calamity."*
(Proverbs 21:23, New International Version)

Maybe you've never been a positive person, and don't feel you can change. Your belief that you can't be positive creates a negative attitude. Whereas if you had a positive belief that you could change, you'd have different attitudes, thoughts, emotions and behavior.

Your emotions that create thoughts lay the foundation for working on the traumas burdening your soul. In my opinion, if the soul isn't free, your physical body can't freely operate in the parasympathetic portion of the body that controls your well-being and vitality.

For example, a 38-year-old war veteran feels he can never forgive himself for all the things he was asked to do during the line of duty. The image below illustrates the kinds of negative self-talk he can have. This destructive cycle of emotions must either be stopped, or his core belief must be changed.

At the core he believes that forgiving himself isn't possible, which isn't true as people vocalize their problems to themselves or to others all the time. But it's the secrets he keeps locked deep inside that make him feel that way.

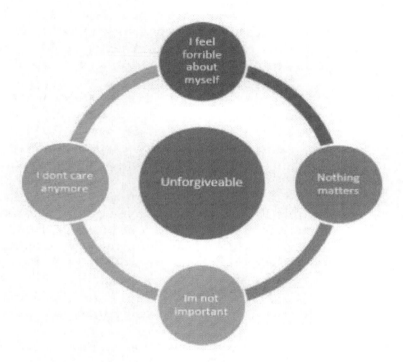

Never underestimate the power of a tiny diagram. Using the one above with my clients (and even people in my life) has brought about new and powerful insights that have shifted their beliefs, attitudes, behavior and thoughts from negative to positive.

*It can work the same for you!*

## Healing Your "Soul Wounds"

The secrets of life, or what I call "soul wounds," will be a big issue while overcoming your traumas. Locked deep inside your soul, they prevent you from exploring your feelings. Your thoughts keep them pushed down so you don't have to deal with difficult or painful issues.

The truth is irrational beliefs of self can, and often will, keep you imprisoned in your trauma, often without you knowing it's occurring. Awareness of and perspective about your condition are important traits to have. Sometimes you need someone you can trust to help you see yourself more clearly.

As you try to internalize the traumas you've experienced, your perspective can become jaded with emotion. Struggling with being objective about your reality, you can become locked in a fight-or-flight mode which compromises your body's health.

In essence, fight-or-flight is when people feel they have little to no control over their brain or their behavior. This can be a very lonely, isolated, physically painful emotional rollercoaster as they can feel removed from the world around them.

Though they might not be able to clearly state what they're experiencing, they nonetheless feel the stress associated with their emotions. Pleasure and joy becomes foreign as they're unable to live in the present, and experience the tangibility of their life. They seek anything to numb the pain (alcohol, drugs, food, sex, gambling, etc.).

Whatever they choose provides a short-term gain with a long-term consequence. An example would be alcohol consumption. Drinking in its early stages might initially help relieve the problem. But then the need to drink more to create the same sense of relaxation and numbness continues the addiction cycle in order to create a feeling of peace.

The next stage is dealing with negative self-beliefs and your pain.

The next stage after that is working on insight and awareness.

The final stage is transformation.

To be fully present, you must be ready for any conversation or emotion that could arise. For example, talking with friends who bring up child abuse could be a trigger for someone who's experienced that kind of trauma.

So try to work out the emotion you placed in the above diagram. This is often done best with honest, loving (and hopefully direct) insight from someone close to you as they can provide a more accurate assessment of how they perceive you.

## Exercise:
## Identifying Your Positive and Negative Emotions

Part of working on your lifestyle changes is being aware of your emotional state of mind.

Because this EMDR technique will help keep you safe during some of the difficult processing, you should be in a calm state of mind for this exercise.

> *"This is the day the Lord has made; We will rejoice and be glad in it."*
> (Psalm 118:24, New King James Version)

- First imagine being by yourself in a peaceful, relaxing place like a beach, a mountaintop, a cabin in the woods, or even your den. For instance, removing myself from my current emotions and state of mind to a lakeshore in the mountains creates a feeling of stillness and tranquility.

- Close your eyes.

- Pay attention to what you're feeling, seeing, sensing and smelling (i.e., pine trees, ocean air, freshly mowed lawn, etc.).

- Allow these new sensations to expand from your core, and become the only ones you're feeling.

After you're done (you'll feel when you should return to your current state), measure how you're feeling on a scale of 1 to 10, where 10 is the most calm. The more you practice this exercise you should easily be able to bring yourself to a 9 or 10 without feeling your trauma or having bad thoughts. Use this exercise any time while processing your emotions to prevent feeling overwhelmed.

Leaving negative emotions unprocessed can create negative core beliefs. Just like you can't see the inside of a basement from the outside of the house, a person can't see their core beliefs just by looking in a mirror. But by going inside themselves and looking around, they can see what needs to be changed.

Referring back to Dr. Brené Brown's "shame research," negative emotions like shame can lead to numerous negative core beliefs. Oftentimes shame can increase fight-or-flight issues, and hinder one's ability to heal.

What emotions did you identify with after doing this exercise?

_____

_____

_____

How long have you been dealing with them? And why?

_____

_____

_____

Have you been avoiding your emotions? _____ Yes _____ No

Do your emotions triggers negative behavior? _____ Yes _____ No

What kinds of negative behavior do your emotions triggers (i.e., drinking, eating, sleeping, suppressing anger, gambling, sex, etc.)? List the emotion(s) and the corresponding activities:

_____

_____

_____

Does one emotion seem to be more debilitating than others (anger, fear, guilt, mistrust, depression, shame, etc.)? _____ Yes _____ No

List any emotions you can identify:

_____

_____

_____

Why are these difficult emotions for you?

_____

_____

_____

I've worked with individuals whose tests showed they had high trauma levels. The higher the trauma level you have, the longer it will take to reprogram your subconscious.

While using frankincense oil with intention and the following affirmation, tell your body to release any trauma causing negative beliefs and emotions in your cells and DNA. (While doing this exercise, remember that it can be a known or unknown trauma.):

(This is from Dr. Mein's book, *Releasing Emotional Patterns With Essential Oils*, that explains the other side of emotions.)

*I choose to release all traumas from all levels of my being that are related to the emotion of_____.*

Be as creative as you want as you can change any of the affirmations I've mentioned to fit your purpose. Doing this exercise several times per day should release or shift your thoughts from negative to positive, or from damaging to constructive.

# Determining Positive Versus Negative Thoughts, Emotions and Feelings

Through this process of honoring your thoughts and feelings, you must *"fix your thoughts on what is true, and honorable, and right, and pure, and lovely, and admirable, Think about things that are excellent and worthy of praise."* (Philippians 4:8, New King James Version)

In other words, what you believe can determine the results of everything you do and receive!

## Thoughts Are Harmonic Energy

Your thoughts are the most prized aspect of your body's vibrational frequency, which is the sum total of your physical, emotional, and spiritual health.

Using the music scale as an example, Dr. Masaru Emoto's work on vibrations with water illustrates this point (more on this in the section "Your Body Electric"). Positive words and thoughts have a stronger vibration, and a more impactful, powerful harmonic.

Simply stated, happy thoughts can protect your body's harmonics. While avoiding emotions and feelings, and saying negative words, can prevent you from overcoming your trauma. Of course you can't live in a state of positivity 24/7. But you can be more mindful of the meaning of the words you speak.

To illustrate this point, I'll use a metaphor of a farmer with seeds (your thoughts) and soil. When a farmer plants seeds in fertile soil (positive feelings), the soil yields bountiful crops. However, no crops can grow if he has fallow or unfertile soil (negative feelings). It's only when fertile soil and healthy seeds align that a perfectly balanced bountiful harvest [your thoughts] can be obtained.

For instance, if you feel you deserve prosperity – but you don't *believe in your heart* you deserve it – you'll plant a fertile seed in rocky soil with little chance of surviving.

Though your body doesn't always know what's going to happen, it knows what vibration goes with what experience.

Think about it this way: Someone cuts in front of you on the freeway. You get angry and swear at them, and your body automatically goes into a fight-or-flight response. Do you need to prepare for a physical battle, such as being attacked by a bear? Of course you don't. Does your body know the difference between a physical attack, or the guy that just cut you off in traffic? No, it doesn't.

*Therefore, it responds the same way to both situations.*

While working with my clients, I place a great deal of importance on what they feel – not just with their mind, but with their entire heart, soul and being. I feel that not believing is why some people heal while others don't.

What you believe – the "prayer of your heart" – is what you'll always receive. Your mind and heart must resonate with each other to begin making powerful changes.

> *"Watch and pray, lest you enter into temptation.*
> *The spirit indeed is willing, but the flesh is weak."*
> (Mark 14:38, New King James Version)

When Jesus's friends were asked to pray for Him, He asked for a short period of sacrifice. But all the hard work and long days of ministry they'd been doing was catching up with them (temptation). Though they were exhausted, they had the desire to pray for him.

While the spirit of a man might willing, his body might not cooperate. For instance, you might have the desire to follow through with your New Year's resolutions. But the temptation to fall back into old habits can be very strong. So this is a powerful proverb by Jesus we can all learn from.

Setting goals is important. Having your goals resonate throughout your complete being will keep you in proper alignment.

Let me reiterate:

### What you *believe in your heart* is the *prayer* you will always receive.

In order for you to experience what you *think* you desire, your *thoughts* and *feelings* have to be in alignment. Until that happens, you'll stay "double-minded" and life will work against you. But once you align your *mind* with your *heart*, you'll become "single-minded" and more focused on your environment and your desires.

## Exercise:
# Assessing Your Thought and Emotional Patterns

This is where you'll write down both positive and negative words you say to yourself and others, as it will help identify the patterns of your thoughts and emotions. A negative mindset is an indicator of deeper emotional issues.

First, you'll learn to understand the emotion and then accept it, thus being able to quickly move past the emotion. Acceptance is the first stage in healing, for without it how can you see your past issues in order to move into the future?

You might not be exactly where you want to be. But where you currently are is okay until you're ready to move to the next stage in your healing.

At this point, you shouldn't be concerned with the words themselves; you just need to get them down so you can think about them. But if they feel overwhelming, take a break and focus your energy on a specific object to re-center your thoughts.

The more focused you become, the clearer your thoughts and attention on what you're thinking. An elevated awareness can alter the cycles and habits of negative thoughts, and create a more positive dialogue in your mind.

Before doing this exercise, you might want to apply a blend of rosewood, spruce, frankincense, and blue tansy oils to both wrists (if you don't have these oils, just use frankincense for balancing). Then hold them against each other until you feel a beat or rhythm, which might take several minutes (this is a great method to help balance your body).

Then you'll want to rub cedarwood oil on both earlobes. Hold each earlobe between a thumb and forefinger until some sort of sensation is felt, which also may take several minutes (I learned this step from Dr. David Stewart in his teachings on courage).

What feelings and heart-centered beliefs arose from this exercise?

_____

_____

_____

_____

_____

What kinds of emotions did you feel? Were you surprised, angry, tentative, in denial, weak, suppressed, etc.?

_____

_____

_____

_____

Based on what you're learning in this book, how do you feel you can strengthen how you handle your emotions?

_____

_____

_____

_____

Based on the earlier farmer metaphor, how do you feel you can increase the "fertility" of your thoughts about yourself not only in your mind, but as you move deeper into your heart?

_____

_____

_____

_____

This exercise will create a change in your body's chemistry and signals. Then your body will grasp the meaning of the words you speak. Because all words create vibrations, you need to eliminate negative thoughts and self-talk from your mental vocabulary.

# Eliminating Negative Thoughts and Self-Talk

Living in a constant state of fear can rob joy and hope from your life. Jason and my stories, plus the case studies, are testimonies that a bright future awaits you even if you're unable to see, feel or believe it at the moment. So letting go, and allowing love and joy come into your life, is one more step on your path to recovery.

Your past can hold you back from everything you've been created for... if you allow it to. You are stronger than you think, so you must learn to invest in yourself by believing your abilities.

## From the Day You Were Born

Entering the world for the first time is a very delicate traumatic process. There are many factors, including the quality of your parents' relationship, your mother's stress level, and the birthing process that affects a fetus before it's born.

A woman's body produces different hormones and neurochemicals based on the emotions she's dealing with during her pregnancy. Therefore, the emotions a fetus experiences are passed on to it by its mother's hormones and neurochemicals.

A great example is the relationship between the child's mother and father. Arguing can increase cortisol levels that can lead to inflammation and increased blood sugar levels that can alter the mother's hormones. Thus, the baby will receive the mother's negative emotions through the blood supply, which can affect its development after it comes into the world.

Emotional issues can be handed down from generation to generation. I've heard many sermons on generational curses, and how sin is handed down through families. This isn't a new concept, but one you must remember as generational emotional issues aren't visible.

## The Genesis of Your Emotions

In the exercise in the chapter on trauma, you determined the emotions you've been feeling and/or avoiding.

Since you've probably been struggling with one or more of them since childhood, there were undoubtedly situations, people, and/or events that helped create your emotional and physical issues. One such consideration is linked to the mother's quality of pregnancy and kinds of traumas during the birth process. Research indicates the different hormones a child is exposed to in its mother's womb could possibly determine the worldview they experience throughout their life.

While in utero, a baby's neural plate receives information based on its mother's hormones and emotional energy within this type of state. Thus causing the infant to be susceptible to a gamut of emotions after it comes into the world. During the first six weeks of life, an infant's circadian rhythms or body clock are also defined. Any alteration in this process can affect brain development and regulation, thereby enhancing the perspective of any traumatic situation.

I'm not saying that a crisis always creates emotional issues. But I believe one of the greatest challenges a human faces is the impact negative emotions can cause.

The point I'm making is removing negative emotions you've gathered during your lifetime (especially ones from your childhood) from your energy field can aid you in your healing process.

I want you to consider the different ways trauma can affect any developmental issue. For instance, some people have a great upbringing and a very pleasant birth process (although I'm finding this is less true with the negative influences the world can have on childbirth), while others unfortunately don't.

## Exercise:
## Holding Your Thoughts Accountable

If you feel like a ship navigating the ocean completely in darkness, or without a rudder to guide you, then you should pay attention to the deeper level of healing you might be needing.

Do you constantly think negative thoughts about yourself?
_____ Yes _____ No

Do you feel like you've always had a negative view of yourself and/or life in general?
_____ Yes _____ No

If you said yes, I want you to pledge to begin changing them into positive ones.

The next time you have a negative thought about yourself, just say "Next!" and make your next thought a positive one (i.e., "My hands are too big" ... "Next!" ... "My hands allow me to build things, do my work, and hold the people I love.") Then write your internal conversation on the lines below.

Negative thought(s):

_____

_____

_____

_____

*NEXT!*

Positive thought(s):

_____

_____

_____

_____

Was this easy or difficult to do? _____ Easy _____ Difficult

Would you be willing to commit to doing this powerful technique for 30 days? If so, over the next month I want you to return to this part of the workbook and write down what you're dealing with. This exercise is powerful, because over the years you can review your notes to see the shifts in your progress.

_____

_____

_____

_____

Holding yourself accountable for your thoughts is important to your recovery. So how do you think you can you be held accountable to prevent backsliding into this bad habit (i.e., do you have an accountability partner to talk to?)?

_____

_____

_____

_____

## CASE STUDY THREE:
### Regaining Self-Worth

It's been questioned if spiritual trauma can cause a physical disease (or vice versa). There are many individuals who believe this concept, as the physical body must get its nourishment from somewhere. However, people can't survive merely on bread and water, as all aspects of their mental, physical, spiritual and emotional well-being need to be nourished.

For example, when my client, Barry, first came to my office, he presented symptoms of not being able to sleep, feelings of loneliness and frustration, and not getting along with people at work and in his personal life.

Constantly becoming irritated by external noise and stimulation, his foggy mind made it difficult to pay attention. His physical symptoms (i.e., a tightness in his chest, and rapid heartbeats) were also becoming more prominent.

Barry stated that though he and his wife weren't at the point of separating, their marriage was struggling. He was worried his relationships with his teenage children were becoming damaged. They didn't want to spend time with him due to his inattentiveness and emotional issues.

Barry had also lost his job. He said that though he hadn't really liked the position much – and that he wouldn't miss his boss or the stress – he was concerned he wouldn't be able to find another one that would pay as well.

Worried about how he and his family would survive, the emotions of fear and shame were becoming overwhelming. Because Barry was full of self-doubt, he said things like he wasn't good enough, and didn't know how things could ever work out. This struck a strong chord with him as he'd been unaware of how much he was dealing with this issue.

While working together, he began to see how frightened he'd become. Feeling these emotions at the surface of his conscious mind felt uncomfortable as he worked toward a new perspective about his life. Knowing the negative tape constantly looping in his unconscious mind had to be re-recorded, he needed to remove any emotional blocks in order to heal (more on how to do this in the workbook chapter, "Energetically Removing Emotional Blocks").

During our sessions, I taught Barry how and where to apply whatever essential oils related to the emotions he was experiencing. A good place to start would be with lavender, frankincense, sage, palo santo, vetiver, neroli, lemon, cedarwood, spruce and ylang ylang.

Then he was given an affirmation to help him begin to "hear' his life (the same affirmation I mentioned earlier from Dr. Mein's book, *Releasing Emotional Patterns With Essential Oils*):

*I choose to release all trauma related to the emotion of* _____ *that no longer serves me.*

The next step was to combine the affirmation and frankincense oil with a light karate chop tap on the base of his skull for about 10 seconds. Barry was asked to do this three times per day to decrease stress and aid in detoxification (see his biophotonic resonance images below to see the results).

The following emotions were the starting point for Barry. There are many others, but these will suffice for this case study:

- shame
- forgiveness
- self-hatred
- betrayal
- loneliness
- abandonment
- acceptance

*NOTE: Kinesiology can also be used to test for emotions that correspond with different parts of the body.*

With her permission, the following tapping points are from Gwenn Bonnell's website, *Tap into Heaven.*

- Governing Vessel-25 (GV-26)
- Conception Vessel-24 (CO-24)
- Stomach-1 (ST-1)
- The other tapping points came from my general understanding: Governing Vessel-20 (connecting the left hand's little finger and thumb to GV-20 and GV-24 while tapping on the back of the neck)
- Governing Vessel-24

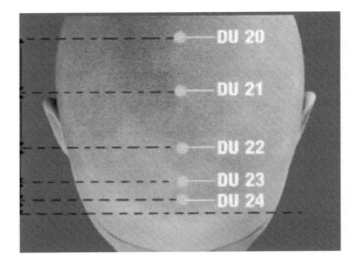

Image adjusted from Full Easy Acupuncture App

- Governing Vessel-6 ( on the image below, count up 4 yellow dots)
- Governing Vessel-8 (on the image below, count up 6 yellow dots)

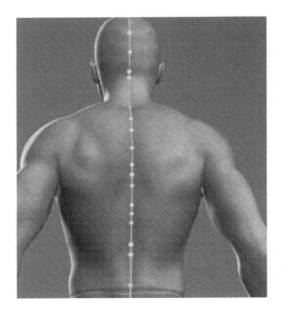

The Biowell images (a gas discharge visual camera) below were used to determine which emotions Barry was struggling with. (Dr. Konstantin Korotkov created the Biowell electrophotonics imaging machine used as a research device. You can learn more about it on his website, korotkov.eu/)

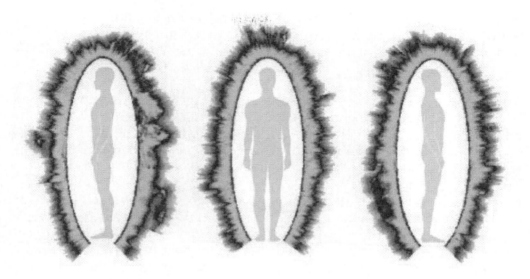

Images used only for educational purposes

I used the Biowell device to take these images that illustrate the disruption of energetic flow throughout Barry's body. A normal or healthy image would have a symmetrical appearance in shape, size, color and appearance.

Barry's energy was stressed, and his vitality was extremely low. His overriding emotions had his focus completely out of whack. I knew he was destined to never overcome his feelings of shame, guilt and fear if he wasn't willing to work on them. So he was given the above affirmation and tapping exercise to treat his trauma between therapy sessions. I also added neurofeedback to retrain his brain's connection networks. (Many people like myself have added remote neurofeedback training to their services.)

During the early sessions I taught Barry Heart Variability Training (HRV), and how to breathe correctly. Connecting his mind and body would decrease the sympathetic lock on his emotions. Breathing properly would also help him learn how to relax.

Through direct-focus activities, HRV showed him how to activate and control his body and mind, and work toward increasing his level of self-regulation. (Heart Math is a great company that offers a very simple approach to HRV for any level of user. Their URL is in References.) Learning to be still and at peace, while clearing his mind and focusing on the positive while allowing him feedback, revealed how well he was able to do this on a scientific level.

With HRV Barry he felt more relaxed and focused. But over time he realized having only the *awareness* of those abilities wasn't enough. At this point much of Barry's trauma was located beyond his consciousness.

As he gained insight into his needs, he strengthened his senses which improved his mental focus muscle, thereby allowing him to control his mind instead of vice versa. In addition to gaining the skills to take control of his life, Barry had learned how to reconnect with his authentic self.

Barry was a terrific "student." The more we got to know each other, the more he opened up about his childhood. He'd been raised to believe that he had to excel in whatever he did. He never felt like he was good enough, so he needed to prove that he was perfect (which created many of his frustrating emotions while his career and marriage was collapsing).

Mirror neurons makes a mother's bonding with her child at birth possible. Your mirror neurons allow you to respond to people's behavior at a cellular level. In other words, you can see people's intentions. For example, when you shake someone's hand your mirror neurons helps you understand the experience of joining hands. This in turn helps create empathy and understanding for that person's world.

However, with poor attachment to their mother during birth, the bonding process might not be fully developed during a child's developmental phases.

This was the case for Barry's childhood. Growing up in a small town where everyone knew everything about everyone, he shared that he'd experienced early childhood trauma. People in the community knew his parents were struggling, and that Barry's mom had had an affair. Due to her own trauma, she lacked the mirror neurons and prefrontal cortex function to help her attach to others and others attach to her. She became distant and married a detached, abusive man.

People didn't know that Barry's father could be violent. Seeking attention elsewhere was his mother's attempt to remove herself from the abusive relationship, while still having someone provide for the family. She kept her husband's physical and emotional abuse well-hidden. So well in fact that when they got a divorce the affair made her look like a bad mother and wife, and her husband like the "good guy." Of course this altered how people viewed and treated the family, which made it difficult for Barry and his siblings to attach and have a sense of belonging in the family.

The further we explored what had happened, Barry said he never wanted to feel that vulnerable or hurt again.

I honed in on his emotions of embarrassment, unworthiness, shamefulness, resentment and pain, and began a discussion of his post-trauma and negative thinking patterns. (In addition to his other affirmations and tapping, I added these to his birth trauma affirmations and emotional block activities.)

Because he diligently did his homework and treatments, Barry felt more relaxed, and began to accept his past and himself. This was the point where I called this his "transition to his spiritual awakening."

Though Barry now feels much better about himself, getting use to his emotions still feels uncomfortable. He reports feeling more in control of his mind and body. It's not taking as long to go to sleep, and he's sleeping much better. His increased self-worth, a greater sense of empowerment, and having more control over his anxieties has greatly enhanced the quality of his relationships and his life in general.

Because Barry is getting along better with his wife and children, he has a deeper connection with them he hadn't felt in the past. Since he can immediately sense any shift in his emotions, he no longer goes into the depths of fight-or-flight like he did in the past.

During my sessions with my clients, one of the biggest challenges to their healing is being transparent about the people in their life. Barry has reported that he's now able to talk about tough situations with his wife, and that he really enjoys their conversations. He said the time spent with her and his children is the most valuable thing in his life.

Previously, Barry had no idea of what he projected to others. But his vibrations shifted the more he worked on healing his emotions (I discuss vibrations in an upcoming chapter). He now has passion for life, smiles more, and is fun to be around.

Overall, life feels really good to Barry. He changed his life by not allowing his problems to consume him. *And you can as well!*

## Exercise:
## Working it Out

It's always good to see things on the other side of the mirror (like Barry needed to do) in case there's something there that reflects what you might be missing, or need to understand with better clarification.

In this exercise, you'll place essential oils on certain areas, then consider the questions ("taking inventory") while the oils are being absorbed into your body.

First, place...

- 2 drops of frankincense oil on your forehead
- 2 drops of juniper oil on top of your head
- 2 drops of palo santo oil on your temples
- 2 drops of cedarwood oil on each earlobe.
- 2 drops of myrrh on your ears.

(You can also use a blend of rosewood, spruce, frankincense and blue tansy oils.)

Then ask the following questions:

What do you need to help ease your current situation?

_____

_____

_____

What techniques you've learned thus far do you feel would be the most helpful?

_____

_____

_____

How often do you feel you'd need to use them (hours, days, months, years?)?

_____

_____

How do you feel that you would be able to tell if you are making progress?

_____

_____

Everything I've discussed so far hinges on you believing these methodologies and essential oils will work. The next chapter focuses on shifting your mindset (your paradigm) to help you see how they can benefit your healing process.

# Shifting Your Mindset About Alternative Holistic Methods

*"People only see what they are prepared to see."*
~Ralph Waldo Emerson

A friend once told me that there's nothing new under the sun. So if you think you've come up something new, you don't know enough about the many achievements of Albert Einstein, ....any's Nobel Prize-winning physicist and scientist, and others like him.

People are constantly searching for ways to help themselves. There are many wonderful developments occurring in today's world of health you don't want to miss. Interestingly, most of them aren't new – they were just before their time.

Some of the methods I discuss are thousands of years old. For example, essential oils aren't new as they date back to biblical times. Their use disappeared during the Dark Ages when ignorance led to persecution of people who used them for healing purposes. But thankfully there was a resurgence during the Renaissance by the physician, Paracelsus, who saw their holistic benefits while treating illnesses.

In other words, changing your mindset from outdated ways of approaching your body's health to alternative methods such as essential oils is what this book is about.

## Reframing Your Paradigm

The word "paradigm" is a modern buzzword. Simply stated, it's a theory or a group of ideas about how something should be done, made, or thought about. Relating to the science of the mind, it's a "set of concepts or thought patterns, including theories, research methods, postulates, and standards for what constitutes legitimate contributions to a field." (*Paradigm,* Wikipedia)

*In other words,* **your mindset determines how you approach your life**.

Have you ever met someone who gave you a warm feeling or "vibe," and you loved being around them? I once met a man whom I wanted to know better as I thoroughly enjoyed being around his energy. I used all my senses to gain insight into why I felt so strongly about wanting to be his friend. And I'm happy to say we're still friends!

*"All elements of the earth have different energies. Some have energy vibrations that whose frequency are very close together, and some have energy vibrations whose frequency are very broad or far apart. In any given matter, the close together the vibrational frequencies, the higher the vibration and the closer that matter is to its energy Source. Or, putting it another way, the more positive the energy of any given matter [including people], the closer the frequencies, and thus, the closer the matter is to its Source.*

*Likewise, the more broad the frequencies of any given matter, the further that energy is from its Source. In other words, the more negative the energy of any given matter, the wider the frequencies, and the further that matter (energy) is from its Source."* (Truman, *Feelings Buried Alive Never Die*; URL in References)

Essential oils are infused with the same chemistry, energy and frequency of plants and herbs created by God.

*This is pretty exciting stuff, so I hope you're excited right along with me!*

## Allowing Your Senses to Guide You

You were born with senses and faculties. One of the greatest ways to increase your level of energy is by fully utilizing your five senses of sight, hearing, taste, smell and touch.

Though I've asked numerous professionals to explain faculties, many aren't able to articulate what they are. Dictionary.com's definitions are faculties are an ability, natural or acquired, for a particular kind of action; one of the powers of the mind, as memory, reason, or speech, an inherent capability of the body (i.e., the faculties of sight and hearing).

As I've previously stated, it's important to get professional medical assistance. But at the end of the day, you need to make an informed decision about your health and your body. Don't just take someone else's word for what you're experiencing. Become educated about your issues, pray on them, explore your five senses and how you feel about your health, and talk to people you trust as they can shed light on your problems you might not have considered.

Throughout your life you've been using your intuition, reason, logic, will, focus and imagination to guide you. These skills can be the most powerful tools in your arsenal of wellness. But you need to constantly sharpen them to prevent them from becoming dulled.

## Increase Your Ability to Focus

For example, you can sharpen your ability to focus to a razor sharp edge. A quick exercise is to hold your index finger in front of your eyes. Make your mind a blank slate, and don't allow any thoughts to enter. Hold your focus and intention solely on your fingertip for three minutes.

At first, you might only be able to stay focused for 20 seconds or so. But the more you do this exercise, the more you'll be able to stay focused for longer periods of time.

## Re-engage Your Imagination

Many people stop using their imagination after puberty as it's considered silly and immature. Of course, dealing with responsibilities is important, especially as you grow older. But that shouldn't overshadow using your creativity. Dreaming about your goals and desires keeps you in touch with your life's purpose.

While growing up, I was always using my senses to do things I shouldn't. For instance, children often daydream during school hours. I loved daydreaming as I took some of the best "trips" during English (which is why I needed a good editor for this book!).

I had big dreams for my life. I told my grandmother that I wanted to cure people. And that when I became a doctor, I could buy her whatever she wanted. I was a very busy boy (at least in my daydreams) envisioning everything I wanted to accomplish when I grew up.

Daydreaming was fine when I was young. But as I got older I lost that ability because I had to make responsible choices about what to do and how to pay for things. The stress of life forced me to be more practical and logical.

One day I finally realized that was the wrong course to have taken. I should have used my senses first, then gain the knowledge to put what I sensed into play (i.e., feeling like I wanted to be a doctor, then going to college to become one).

But then I also realized I had lost my ability to daydream so I could learn to use the skills God had given me. It was an invaluable lesson to learn that everyone has more talent and ability they'll ever be able to develop.

Learning to use all five of your senses and faculties can alter your state of vibration and consciousness by shifting negative energy to positive. Believing in yourself will give you the motivation to fight for your life with increased vigor and determination on a deeper subconscious level.

Utilizing your senses to release trauma allows you to be in the present. Not staying in the moment keeps you stuck in the past, or throws you into a questionable future where you'll continue to guard yourself against growth. Utilizing all of your senses will require you to accept any emotions or thoughts you're feeling, and let go of any defensiveness.

A good blend of essential oils to heighten your senses is...

- 20 drops of frankincense
- 14 drops of onycha
- 14 drops of myrrh
- 8 drops of juniper
- 5 drops of clove
- 3 drops of cinnamon
- 3 drops of cedarwood
- 3 drops of rosemary
- 3 drops of helicrysum

You can blend this in a larger amount, or leave it as listed. Or you can blend other oils you might prefer better. You can take the larger amount with you and use it all day.

Clove and cinnamon are considered "hot oils," so use them sparingly in the beginning. The more often you use them in smaller amounts, the more tolerant you'll become. If you don't like the smell of any individual oils, or after they're blended, you can do the "smell affirmation."

# Exercise:
## Connecting to Your Senses

This very simple but important exercise helps shift your paradigm so you can recognize which sense is being used at what time. Then if it's the wrong sense (i.e., using sight when you should be using touch or smell), you'll automatically shift to the correct one.

Which of your senses do you feel are the strongest? And why?

_____

_____

_____

_____

Are there times you were aware of something, but couldn't pinpoint exactly what it was? _____ Yes _____ No

If yes, explain the situation, and what generated your particular response (i.e., fear of dying, didn't know where to go, didn't want to upset someone, couldn't pinpoint the emotion you were feeling, etc.):

_____

_____

_____

_____

Which of your senses mentioned above do you feel are your strongest? And why?

_____

_____

_____

_____

Do you feel stressed? _____ Yes _____ No

Has trauma affected your ability to use your senses? _____ Yes _____ No

If yes, which stress and/or trauma is having a stronger effect? And why?

_____

_____

_____

_____

Commit to using affirmations, tapping, and your oil blend for the next 30 days to help you break old habits, and use your senses and faculties more often.

I've discussed many different ways to treat your conditions. Now I'm going to show you how to utilize affirmations and essentials oils with the power of tapping.

# Controlling Your Thoughts and Emotions with Tapping

*"A man's spirit sustains him in sickness,*
*but a crushed spirit who can bear?"*
(New King James Version, Proverbs 18:14)

Jeremiah 29 states "'For I know the plans I have for you,' declares the Lord. 'Plans to prosper you and not to harm you. Plans to give you hope and a future."

One of the benefits of the aroma from essential oils is everyone gets the opportunity to enjoy them. One day when I was talking to a friend in a retail store, one of her friends (who doesn't know what I do) said she had a headache and was tired. My friend (I'll call her Dawn) tends to be very "essential oily," so a strong aroma was very present that I could work with.

When I asked Dawn's friend if she wanted to quickly get rid of her headache, she answered, "Yes. But I don't know what could do that." Because there a scent was already present, I didn't need to open a bottle to conduct a measurement.

Taking a quick inventory of her issues, I sensed her liver and pancreas weren't functioning correctly, and that her stomach was upset. I instructed her to inhale and count to three while I worked on nine points on her body and head to bring them back into balance with each other.

When I asked her how her head felt, she looked at me and said, "It's the weirdest thing. It doesn't both me any more."

Believe it or not, using your senses for situations like this is really that easy.

Because of the kind of work I do, I know the places on a person's body that can respond to treatments. For instance, sensing changes in people's electrical activity can help their body make the necessary shifts.

One such avenue is to learn how to shift your energy to alter your emotional and/or psychological states to shift your physiological conditions.

## The Altered State of Thoughts and Emotions

Thoughts can have a trickle-down effect on people. Since they're a very powerful source of energy, they can shift in many different dimensions. For example, reading this book could shift your mindset, which in turn would affect people around you and people around them ad infinitum.

*"Therefore, thought as matter is impossible to destroy. Feelings as energy, or matter, are also impossible to destroy. Nevertheless, matter can be altered. Consequently, the energy of feelings and of thoughts can be changed. If the feeling or the thought is negative matter (energy) it can be changed to positive matter (energy)."* (Truman, *Feelings Buried Alive Never Die*)

The world of energy can be changed by belief, faith and quantum physics. While growing up in a small Texas town, going to church every Sunday and Wednesday was a fact of life. I believed everything in the Bible, and what I was taught in Sunday School.

Though God had a plan for me to do something different with my life, He needed me to stay grounded in my spiritual beliefs. He taught me a great deal through my teens. But I went through an early metamorphosis during my first year of college where I faced possible misdemeanor charges for my poor choices and behavior.

When I called my parents to tell them what happened, I was taken aback by their lack of response. My family has a history of not dealing with issues, which affected my feeling of imperfection. Since everything always had to look perfect, this situation brought shame to the forefront, which I didn't know how to handle.

This was when I really started seeking spiritual enlightenment. I went to a Christian college where I dug deeper into my faith and relied on having Christ in my life.

The relationship with my father wasn't great. But I knew he loved me because he attended my high school sporting events when he wasn't passionately tending the farm. Because I wanted a closer relationship with him, I'd try to strike up a conversation, no matter how awkward I felt, just so we could talk. I loved hearing stories his friends told about things they'd done together because it kept me connected to him.

I'm mentioning this as it set the tone for my spiritual relationship with my Heavenly Father. From my experience with my Earthly father, I learned that although men could be distant, they were there for me when I needed them. This was exactly the relationship I had with God.

*"The most profound blessing our spirit needs to receive and can receive is the father-heart of God, His special creation of us, his kind intention toward us, His matchless love for us, His glory revealed in us."*
(Burk, *Blessing Your Spirit*, 2009)

It's fascinating how the Lord works out all of the details of one's life. All they need to do is pay attention.

After I got married, I still had a lot of work to do on my spirituality. While practicing as a licensed professional, I was also active in my church's youth group. One summer I went to camp with the group for a mountaintop experience. Along the way, one of the leaders got a call that her son was just diagnosed with cancer.

Because the trip started off emotionally difficult, I had no idea my own emotional "cancer" would be dealt with as well. Having God move in me while leading a group of young men was a life-altering experience. The youth leader was completely blown away when I opened up to him about what the Lord was designing for me.

When I called my wife to tell her everything that was going on, she said, "I always knew there were issues. Why hadn't you opened up to me about them before now?"

Telling no one was exactly the problem I'd been having. My shame had become overwhelming, so much so the trauma of it led me to withdrawal and periodic depression.

Never wanting to talk about the past kept me in a constant state of emotional bondage and numbness about the past. Though I yearned to be around people, I distanced myself from them and became socially awkward. Because I couldn't connect with myself in order to connect with others, this is where I began my transformation.

I can't say things have been perfect since that glorious day I revealed my problems to my wife, and those who are close to me. But I can say they've been much better. Today my life is wonderful. I'm blessed beyond belief that I have the best family a guy could ask for, and that I can thoroughly enjoy the moments I have with myself and others.

*"A cheerful heart is good medicine,*
*but a crushed spirit dries up the bones."*
(Proverbs 17:22, New King James Version)

I had just starting using essential oils at the time all of this occurred. It's my firm belief that God gave me His "medicines" to help me walk through my journey of self-discovery.

My counseling practice also changed. I began to explore what really helped people, and trying to uncover the issues instead of just diagnosing the symptoms.

My early experiences of using essential oils with spirituality is beyond words. Every experience moved me closer to the world of energy healing, which is what I'm currently practicing with myself and my clients.

My experiences also created my strong thirst for knowledge. If the Lord wouldn't have been guiding me on my path, I don't think I would have ever found the energy movement. Having the knowledge and education to heal people's emotional issues is the foundation on which I built my practice.

*Now, that's something to be really excited about!*

I'm sharing this story to help you understand that trauma happens to everyone.

Looking back on my life, I see the Lord's healing and understanding through vibration. I now understand that when He speaks, things happen. Though I don't understand how it happened, it makes sense that He created the world by speaking it.

Watching the exciting world of energy movement help people feel better, I wanted to learn more about how it worked. Because essential oils had so many different uses, I asked the Lord to show me how I could use them personally and in my practice. The creativity for their many uses He gave me was just incredible!

Of course God can heal you without any of this. From personal experience, I lacked the belief and faith that God heals. I had prayed for healing many times, but felt nothing.

*But once I believed that healing could occur, it did!*

## Life is Right Before Your Eyes

Emotions can be very deceiving. Looking back on my life, I know my prayers weren't answered in the way I wanted. But in the way that was right for my life's journey.

Because I live in the windiest city in America, I've witnessed the destruction wind can cause. You can't see wind, but you can feel it. Just like I never allowed feeling my emotions until I felt safe, and was ready to begin healing.

> *"To every thing there is a season,*
> *and a time to every purpose under the heaven."*
> (Ecclesiastes 3, New King James Version)

That was a very enlightening season for me. An amazing time when I began to feel the Lord move within me. A time when I began to understand His design for my life. A time when I asked for healing with a spirit of receiving, just like receiving gifts from others.

Arthur Burk's book, *Blessing Your Spirit,* is full of incredible resources, including a 21-day blessing for your spirit. Doing all 21 days early in your healing process will help you understand more about your life's purpose.

As an example...

Day 1:

_____[fill in your name]_____, I call your spirit to attention in the name of Jesus of Nazareth *(listen with your spirit to hear God's words)* "for you created my innermost being; you knit me together in my mother's womb. I praise you because I am fearfully and wonderfully made; your works are wonderful, I know that full and well. My frame was not hidden from you when I was made in the secret place. When I was woven together in the depths of the earth, your eyes saw my unformed body. All the days ordained for me were written in your book before one of them came to be." (Psalm 139:13-16)

_____[fill in your name]_____, your Father made you special. You are a very special person, created and crafted and designed by God your Father. Before the foundation of the world, your Father planned for you. You are no accident. You did not have to exist, but your Father willed you into existence. He chose the day and the time you would start your life. (Burk, 2009)

I'm not comparing unseen electrical fields to the Lord. But being led to understand the unseen in a new way deepened my belief they work. In other words, I no longer needed to see something in order to believe in it.

I also realized my clients no longer needed the emotions associated with their traumas. So I began using different devices and modalities with them, and the results came quicker and faster. This was an exciting time because I was learning so much. And I'm still learning every single day!

What I'm discussing probably wouldn't be taught in mainstream education. But everyone should be a good steward for their body in a society that only sees healthcare as a billion-dollar industry.

If anything I say sounds weird, or makes you feel uncomfortable, learning how to use all of your senses will increase your faith and belief that it's all possible. Praying on it will also help you handle your emotions differently so you can have a healthier, happier life.

## Getting in Touch with the Real You

*"Believe in yourself! Have faith in your abilities!*
*Without a humble but reasonable confidence in your own powers*
*you cannot be successful or happy."*
~Norman Vincent Peale

During my research over the years, I found that most people don't need to be told what to do. They just need to identify the emotions that create negative behavior or energy. They need to be educated about what tools will work to harness positive energy and release the negative.

To be in the present, you must accept whatever emotions arise. People have many emotions related to past events. Because they don't think about about them on a regular basis (or at all), they think they're permanently gone while they're actually lying dormant.

A situation isn't alive when it has no emotional negative response attached to it. But if a situation still has an emotional response, you can begin to clear it energetically to permanently remove the emotion.

*Though change isn't easy, you can do anything if you believe in yourself.*

Since the skills you'll learn in this workbook can be very powerful, I'd like to encourage you to get in touch with the "real" you.

It's my aim to teach you the difference between negative and positive emotions and feelings, the difficulties you struggle with, and how to utilize your new skills to your benefit.

I know this might feel a bit too "touchy feely." But please hang in there with me as this is where the stages of change are crucial to your healing.

*"Emotions and feelings are often thought of as being one and the same. Although they are related, there is a difference between emotions and feelings, and they both serve you in their own unique way.*

*The difference is important because the way you behave in this world is the end result of your feelings and emotions. Feelings express your true identity, while emotions reveal how you have been taught to respond to events in your life.*

*Learning the difference between feelings and emotions is crucial in understanding ourselves and initiating personal long-term change. Experts in many fields of behavior agree that our deep feelings come from an unchanging belief about life that holds our identity together, while our emotions are purely physically based, subject to change and are basically reactions to life events."* (Voris, *Difference Between Emotions and Feelings*, 2009)

Simply stated, a physical condition can be caused or intensified by a psychological factor, such as stress, anxiety, depression, etc. Clinical research is helping people understand how emotions affect their body and vice versa.

The pain of trauma can create the desire to turn to anything such as alcohol, drugs, food, sex, etc., that numbs emotions. Like a light switch you can turn off and on, a part of your brain turns off to prevent feeling or remembering pain.

However, I believe it must be turned back on in order to heal. Gaining new insight into your emotions will change the way you interact with the rest of the world. It will allow you to stay out of sympathetic lock, and in a healthier state of parasympathetic release (discussed later).

# Tapping to Release Stress, Tension and Anxiety

*"In every culture and in medical tradition before ours,*
*healing was accomplished by moving energy."*
~Albert Szent-Gyorgyi (1960)

Tapping is a powerful tool used by millions of people to help them become centered, calm and focused. Healing through touch and other means has been used for centuries. Even early Christians used the laying on of hands through prayer.

A study by Dr. John Zimmerman using a squid magnetometer, a device that detects very microscopic amounts of currents in the body's electrical field in order to measure how touch therapy affects humans.

*"The therapeutic touch signal pulsed at a variable frequency, ranging from 0.3 to 30 Hz, with most of the activity in the range of 7-8 Hz. In other words the signal emitted by the practitioner is not steady or constant, it 'sweeps' or 'scans' through a range of frequencies."* (Zimmerman, "The Era of Energy Medicine")

Tapping (aka: EFT, Emotional Freedom Technique) is thought of as a form of "psychological acupressure" where you use your fingertips on specific places on your head, chest and pulse points to balance your energy. It helps creates physical and emotional relief as you think about then release problems. It can remove pain, food cravings and negative emotions, and increase positivity to help you achieve your goals.

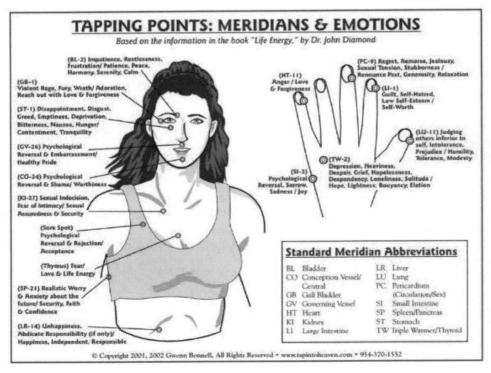

Usage granted by Gwenn Bonnell

One of the very first tapping exercises I did was with a businessman who wanted to control stress in his personal and business lives. When I showed him how to tap while applying essential oils, to his surprise he noticed an instant difference in how he was feeling.

As quoted from *The Tapping Solution* website:

*"[Tapping] can be used with specific emotional intent towards your own unique life challenges and experiences. Most importantly, it gives you the power to heal yourself, putting control over your destiny back into your own hands.*

*In recent years there's been a growing pool of undeniable research that proves what millions of people all over the world over have known for some time now: that EFT produces real, lasting breakthroughs and significantly improves or even eliminates conditions that hospital treatments, medication and years of psychotherapy often fail to adequately deal with.*

*Studies done at no less than Harvard Medical School verify these assertions. Research done at the prestigious university during the last decade found that the brain's stress and fear response – which is controlled by an almond-shaped part of your brain called the amygdala – could be lessened by stimulating the meridian points used in acupuncture, acupressure, and of course, tapping.*

*Although these studies focused on acupuncture and as such, used needles, follow-up double-blind research revealed that stimulating the points through pressure, as we do in tapping, gave rise to a similar response!"*

Another exciting research project was undertaken by Dr. Dawson Church whose team performed a randomized controlled trial to study how an hour-long tapping session would impact the stress levels of 83 subjects [Dawson, EFT Tapping].

After the session was over, Dr. Church and his team measured their level of cortisol (a hormone secreted by the body when it undergoes stress). Their findings were the average level of cortisol reduction was 24%, with a whopping reduction of almost 50% in some subjects. In comparison, there was no significant cortisol reduction in those who underwent an hour of traditional talk therapy.

Dr. Church also created The Stress Project that teaches tapping to war veterans suffering from PTSD. The results have been astounding: there was an average 63% decrease in PTSD symptoms after six rounds of tapping.

If you find it hard to change things on the physical realm, tapping might help by reaching your subconscious realm.

Having mentioned Stanley Burroughs earlier in the section on cleansing the inside of your body, he also created and coined the term "Vita-Flex" in his book titled, *Healing for the Age of Enlightenment.*

Burroughs refers to Vita-Flex as "a complete system of internal body 'controls'." To paraphrase, when properly applied to the appropriate control points, a vibrational, healing energy is released to relieve pain, and remove the symptoms as well as the causes of illness. This reflex system encompasses the entire body and mind, and releases all kinds of tension, congestion, and maladjustments.

Below is a chart showing all the points where essential oils can be best utilized:

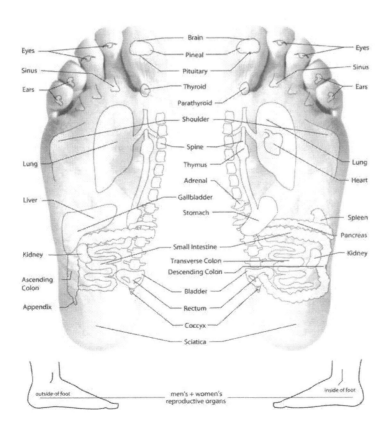

(It's not my intention to discuss the full scope of Vita-Flex. But you can visit the CARE website at raindroptraining.com for classes that might be taught near you. The depth of knowledge you'll gain from the CARE experience would be an excellent complement to the techniques you're learning.)

During their initial session, I've had addicts say they feel similar to when they're under the influence of a substance, like alcohol or drugs. To me this translates as a euphoric state of relaxation and enjoyment in which they don't have any other state to compare it to.

Sometimes peoples don't feel anything, which is fine as not everyone does their first time. However, every time I test a person's aesthetic layers (the energy field surrounding the outer parts of the body), the feeling reveals itself as a negative belief. This indicates their emotional state needs to be shifted, and that a positive change is occurring.

No matter how small a shift might be, the unconscious part of the brain is well aware it's occurring. For example, when you meet someone, you either love them or don't want to be around them. Their vibration in your unconscious brain led you to those feelings.

All signs indicate this trend of revealing positive results will sway skeptics as millions of people around the globe continue to discover the power of tapping.

# Exercise:
# Using Essential Oils and Tapping to Finally Have the Peace You've Been Longing For!

*Determining Your Stress Level...*

Before you begin this exercise, on a scale of 0 to 10 (10 being the highest) write down the stress level you're experiencing at this very moment: _____

Then ask yourself what stressors you're dealing with, and what might have caused them (identifying them before you begin tapping directs energy to the right places in your body). It's fine if you can't identify any or all at this point. Just do your best.

_____

_____

_____

Doing this tapping method several times per day will help balance the frequency between your brain, heart, and body. It will control your emotions, which will allow you to feel calmer and clearer. (I often have clients report incredible changes by using this exercise. So the more you do it, the better you'll feel!)

The Oils:

Apply either bergamot, frankincense, myrrh, spruce, lavender, peppermint or vetiver (or a combination of any of these) from the tip of your nose... up your forehead to the top of your head... then down the back of your head, your neck and spine all the way down to the base of your tailbone (your electrical "control center").

(I highly recommend the blend I mention after Bonnell's Tapping Procedure chart below. If you haven't purchased all the oils, free to use any of the single ones above. Many people report success with both singles or a blend.)

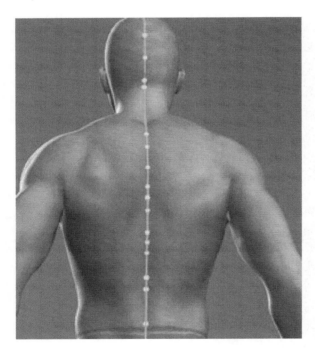

The Tapping:

• With your right hand, tap the back of your head where your spine meets your skull with a light, soft "karate chop." This kind of tapping activates the cerebral cortex, and is the motion you'll use for most tapping techniques I'll be describing.

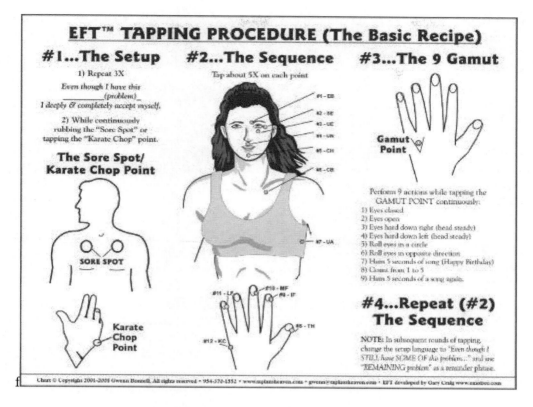

Usage granted by Gwenn Bonnell

Feel free to utilize Gwenn's incredible steps as well as the the ones below. The oils will also help with the tapping.

- This slightly modified blend you can use with tapping combines the oils Egyptians used for emotional clearing:

  - 20 drops frankincense
  - 14 drops onycha
  - 14 drops myrrh
  - 8 drops juniper
  - 5 drops clove
  - 3 drops cinnamon
  - 3 drops cedarwood
  - 3 drops rosemary
  - 3 drops helicrysum

If you choose to use individual oils, just place a few drops into the palm of your hand, stir with a fingertip, then apply as needed.

- Place your left index figure on your right temple. Rub clockwise in circles for about 20 seconds with your eyes open, and then 20 with your eyes closed. Then repeat for the left temple.

  Remember to inhale for 6 seconds and exhale for 8 seconds while rubbing in clockwise circles. Have the intention of tapping on the hypothalamus and thalamus in your brain.

- Then place vetiver oil on your chest over your heart and on the middle of your forehead. Vetiver is photosensitive, meaning in the sunlight it can quickly cause a burn or blister. So it's best to do this in a place with minimal light.

  To heighten electrical activity in your brain and heart, place your left hand over your heart and your right hand on top of your head. Use a light karate chop tapping for about 30 seconds.

- Then tap your heels together (this is the same kind of tapping you use on the back of your neck) for about 30 seconds.

What kinds of physical and/or emotional responses did you notice while doing this exercise?

_____

_____

_____

If you didn't notice anything, put a drop of frankincense on each wrist, then hold them together. Inhale deeply and wait for a light tingling sensation or pulse. Until you feel it, try to keep your mind empty of thoughts.

One you feel the tingling, scan your body slowly from the top of your head down to the bottom of your toes. Pay close attention to your senses. What did you feel while doing this?

_____

_____

_____

This exercise seems to be more difficult for men. It's not a feminine issue; it's about how they've been raised and taught to deal with emotions. Rough-and-tumble play has its place. But being in touch with your senses will increase your well-being, your athleticism, stamina and brain power.

## Additional Application

I'd like to suggest that you do this additional application to make the experience even more powerful. If possible (and I hope it is), follow the above oil/tapping session with several drops of oil of patchouli, cypress, orange, ylang ylang, lavender or frankincense to the top of your head with the intention of holding on to the transformation you've begun.

### To help boost your endocrine system...

The endocrine system controls growth and development, reproduction, metabolism and homeostasis (your body's internal balance) through a network of glands that produce, store and secrete hormones.

Here I'll focus on your adrenal glands that produce a variety of hormones including adrenaline, and the steroids aldosterone and cortisol (that causes stress). Imbalanced adrenal glands can cause all sorts of issues, such as difficulty getting out of bed, chronic fatigue even after you wake up, a foggy mind, or finishing your tasks during the day.

The Oils:

Oils that work well are nutmeg, ginger, spearmint, myrtle, fennel and anise.

Place 1, 2, 3 or even more drops of a single oil, or a blend of the oils (sometimes it smells so good you'll want a little more) over the adrenal area above each kidney. You can also put them on the soles of your feet, as the feet have large pores and can quickly absorb the oils.

Then place more oil in the palm of your non-dominant hand, and stir it clockwise several times. This activates the oil, then places it on the area around the kidneys in the lower parts of your back. Hold the intent of what you are doing in your mind and continue.

The Tapping:

- As previously mentioned, your adrenal glands sit on top of both of your kidneys. Tap that area on the left side of your with your fingers, while tapping at the base of your neck and skull with your right hand. I like to use the location of the neck and skull often as it activates the prefrontal cortex (the executive center) to communicate more effectively.

- You can also put 2 to 8 drops of oil into the well of your hand, and stir it clockwise. Then apply the oil to your entire abdomen which will help the energetic needs of the fight-or-flight response.

## To help your pituitary...

The pituitary is activated by the amino acid, thyrotropin from the hypothalamus, which in turns activates your thyroid. Your thyroid makes the hormone thyroxine to furnish the molecule ATP (adenosine triphosphate) to the mitochondria of your body. This is your body's natural process that become disrupted.

The Oils:

Oils that work well for this tapping procedure are vetiver, bergamot, frankincense, ylang ylang, patchouli, clove, peppermint, spruce, valerian and lemon. You can use them individually, or blended together.

Apply the oil(s) from the tip of your nose over the top of your head down your spine to the belt line.

Then place a couple drops of one or more oils into the well of your left hand. Stir it several times with your left index fingertip while praying about/focusing on your pituitary. Then use that same fingertip to apply it to your body in the same manner.

The Tapping:

- Place your left index finger in the center of your forehead with the intention of helping the pituitary.

- With this intention, the process might need to be slowed or speeded up.

- Since balance is the key intention, tapping the back of your skull with with your right fingertips (remember – a light karate-type tapping), while placing your left index finger on the center of your forehead, will help balanced your system.

  Tap for about 15 seconds, or until you sense a slight or subtle shift in energy. While doing this exercise, inhale as you count to 5, then breathe out as you count to 5. Be patient if you don't sense anything in the beginning. You can't ruin the process if you hold on to your intention for healing.

- Then move your left index fingertip to the top center of your head, and repeat the same steps.

- Then move your left index fingertip down the left side of your head to just above your ear (the temporal lobe that's responsible for memory and other tasks). Repeat the same steps as above.

- Then move your left index fingertip to the right side of your head just above your ear to the right temporal lobe. Repeat the same steps.

- Then move your left index fingertip to the center of the back of your head to just about where the spinal cord enters the skull. This might tough to tap with this point as you're touching and tapping in very similar regions. Just do your best.

After you've finished tapping, on a scale from 0 to 10 what is your stress level at this point? _____

Can you tell a difference in your state of being? _____ Yes _____ No

Explain either response:

_____
_____
_____
_____
_____

Since there are many advanced methods of tapping and linking systems together, this is only an introduction for the purpose of this book. There's a great deal of information on the Internet and in libraries, so I'd like to encourage you to find out as much as possible about this valuable wellness tool.

For example, further information and a chart on tapping points can be found at either The Tapping Solution or Tap into Heaven websites (URLs in References).

# The Science of Surviving

Every person's life is grounded in the physical, emotional, psychological and even ethereal components of surviving that can often be a tumultuous existence.

I love that modern-day science plays a fundamental part in people's lives. But I'm often reminded of primitive camping trips I've enjoyed over the years. (People who've been in the military can identify with the word "primitive" as it means using only the minimal tools from a pack necessary to survive a multi-day trip.)

The tools can vary based on your knowledge and skills. Because I'm not a big guy, I can't carry the weight more muscular men can. For my first camping trip, I over-packed as though I was going "car camping." Trust me, it wasn't fun carrying all that equipment over twelve miles up then back down the side of a mountain.

But as my skills grew over time, I learned what was essential to have a more positive camping experience. While walking trails through the mountains, I connected with nature by studying the vegetation and the environment. By becoming immersed in the experience, instead of struggling against it, I learned a great deal about myself.

## Stress is Nothing to Ignore

While worrying about how to pay your bills, feeling road rage while in traffic, or while having arguments at work or disagreements with your spouse, etc., your stress threshold becomes and stays very high.

If you don't learn how to control your stress, that high level becomes your default. It can create physical issues such as muscle tension, hypertension, diabetes and emotional issues that can damage and/or destroy your relationships at home and at work.

Combining the experience of the stillness on those camping trips with other life experiences taught me how to be still. I learned to exist in the present with my surroundings while clearing my mind so I could enjoy the moment of silence. It's an essential survival skill I'm grateful to have learned.

Being in nature was also where I began to experience the more ethereal and spiritual aspects of my being. I learned that the body is much more than just chemistry, because God created everything to be in balance. When life is out of balance, your body will communicate what's wrong if you know how to be still and listen to what it's saying.

Understanding your body and your surroundings, while working to better yourself and helping those around you as you become stronger, is one of the greatest skills utilized in neuroplasticity.

## Neuroplasticity: Your Mind's "Wiring"

As a psychotherapist, I'm in awe of the science behind the mind/body experience of physical and psychological trauma. The theory of neuroplasticity (how the plasticity or adaptability of the brain and neural connections) has been around for many years:

*"It's believed that an American named William James presented the first theory of neuroplasticity around 120 years ago in his book Principle of Psychology. This psychologist and philosopher is widely credited with first suggesting that the human brain is capable of reorganizing.*

*Although William James was the first person to have mentioned the brain could reorganize, the first documented person known to use the term Neuroplasticity was a Polish Neuroscientist named Jerzy Konorski in 1948. Konorski suggested that over time neurons that had coincidental activation due to the vicinity to the firing neuron would after time create plastic changes in the brain."* (History of Neuroplasticity)

Today's search to understand how the mind and body work together is a fast-growing field in neuroscience, which should be exciting for individuals suffering from a traumatic brain injury (TBI), stroke, OCD, anxiety, depression, addiction, and numerous others ailments and conditions.

Researchers in the field of neuroplasticity are proving how neural connections can be "remade," so to speak. For instance, from his Taub Therapy Clinic at the University of Alabama, Dr. Edward Taub teaches brain-injured individuals how to retrain their brain and regain motor skills and sensory integration.

To get to that point, he analyzed numerous different brain maps and research projects to understand how the brain and nervous system is wired. Then he ascertained what he could do to help traumatized individuals regain connectivity.

His patients suffering from brain injury disconnection have experienced incredible results.

*"Taub Therapy gives patients hope that they can recapture the life they had before suffering a stroke or TBI."* ~Edward Taub, Ph.D.

## A Relaxed Person is a Healthy Person

Through my Heart Rate Variability training (HRV), I learned that a relaxed person is a healthy person. Working through the olfactory center (the sense of smell) of the cerebral cortex, essential oils quickly go to work to shift a negative state to a positive state of feeling calm and relaxed.

*Knowing your brain can change through neuroplasticity, and that you're not stuck with your symptoms, should be very good news!*

Because of my love for nature, it made sense to incorporate a natural approach to understanding myself. My senses weren't quite as strong while learning how to camp in the mountains. But through neuroplasticity, I've gained an understanding of the wisdom that lies within my body that helped me become stronger in all areas of my life.

Your perspective will be challenged during your wellness efforts, which might create a bit of chaos in your thinking. But this is an excellent opportunity to shift old thoughts (paradigms) to new ones, which will help you live the life you deserve!

## Neurochemicals and Drugs

Your mental abilities include your imagination, will, reason, logic and intuition. (Intuition is very important as it boosts your imagination, which in turn increases hope.) Creativity is also important, because without it you can lose purpose and hope.

Neurochemicals in your nervous system regulate your thoughts and emotions. Depending on well they're balanced, they can have a profound effect on how you feel and function, and your moods and behavior.

Pharmaceutical drugs attempt to assist the body by regulating chemicals. For example, if your body can't produce dopamine, certain medications can block receptor sites to fool your body into feeling it's had enough.

If you stop the medication, your body doesn't know dopamine production is low, so it has to try to increase it. By this time the symptoms will have returned, so healing will take longer.

"Street drugs" such as a heroine or methamphetamines eventually become addictive and troubling. Sadly, death is very possible. The substance works to stop the body's natural process, which creates a dependence on the drug as the body can no longer properly function.

Even high-risk behaviors, and an imbalance within the body, can be created through the release of adrenaline and neurochemicals.

Before turning to any kind of synthetic chemical-laden drug, understanding the issues your body is facing can be done via blood work, hair analysis, energetic analysis, and many others kinds of evaluations.

I understand that sometimes prescribed drugs are a necessary part of a treatment protocol. But you need to have a solid wellness plan (hopefully one that includes holistic alternatives such as essential oils) in place other than purely relying on drugs to make you feel better.

Regardless of whether you're considering using a pharmaceutical drug, or an alternative form of medicine, you might want to first seek a professional such as a homeopath or naturopath (or a therapist such as myself) well-versed in minerals, amino acids, vitamins and hormones. They will holistically assess your problems so they can prescribe the correct tests to fine-tune a wellness plan.

I'd like to suggest finding the right professional who won't come up with an immediate diagnosis, then prescribe a set of protocols or treatments typical for that diagnosis. So look for one who will fully assess your symptoms, then take the time to educate you about various methods beneficial to your particular problem.

(Unfortunately, I don't find this approach to be very common among today's medical practitioners. But combining alternative methods such as essential oils with Western medicine is steadily growing, as the benefits are becoming more evident.)

Your body must be supported no matter what you're dealing with. For example, race cars run better by using high octane fuel sources. The driver doesn't question the car must have gas to run.

It's the same with your body as it needs the basic essentials to function. It's just finding the right "fuel" to keep it running on all cylinders.

Dr. Hawkins (veritaspub.com) created a calibration level of emotions from 1 to 1,000. For example, an individual who's dealing with PTSD might experience all or most of the negative emotions at the bottom of the list. However, if they can work towards the 200 level calibration, a sense of courage and affirmation can be obtained.

I've used Dr. Hawkins's method to determine how fight-or-flight, stress and developmental issues keeps my clients locked in a lower emotional calibration that affects their entire vibration. For instance, stress can trigger certain emotions. If a person is stuck at a level of, say, guilt (a calibration of 30) or shame (a calibration of 20), they won't be able to tap into adequate coping skills to maintain their emotional stability. They lose hope that they'll never be able to overcome their issues.

Many clients initially come into my office with a very low calibration under 100. But they're often reach the higher level calibration of courage at 200. As they remove their emotional numbness, they become more integrated in all aspects of their being. So moving the calibration higher has served its purpose.

As they say, 'pride goeth before the fall.' Courage, or a 200-level calibration, is where change really begins to occur. The calibration level of 200 is just above the calibration level of pride at 175, which would keep individuals struggling with an addiction, trauma or other major issue stuck in the cycle.

Dr. Hawkins makes the argument that staying stuck at the "pride" level perpetuates a person's negative cycle of behavior. He also believes that it's easy for people to get in and stay stuck in the addiction cycle.

Emotions are tricky. When a person feels better, they feel pride in their accomplishments. But not advancing to the level of courage can continue old behavior patterns, so they should try to rise above the level lower in order to achieve their full potential.

*Many people have done it, and you can too!*

I've found the major difference between clients who become well versus those who don't is the level of developmental trauma and the individual's level of belief. They might be facing numerous overwhelming issues that make them feel there's no end in sight.

But individuals who possess faith and belief that certain treatments work (such as essential oils and the treatments I use) will invest time and energy in their wellness. (I realize I often discuss belief and faith.

But they really are one of the most powerful tools to have in your arsenal of wellness.)

For my clients experiencing issues such as self-doubt or recrimination, their emotional blocks must be removed in order to boost their levels of faith and belief.

Though the inner struggles of each individual are different, everyone has the ability to make it to the same destination. When you lack passion, belief, faith, or motivation, you must take a deep personal inventory. People who take the time for self-reflection often find the blocks that are holding them back.

## Additional Tools to Have in Your Wellness Arsenal

Following is a list of things that can help you reach a higher level of awareness:

- Purchase then incorporate essential oils into your daily routine by putting them on your skin.
- Combine the oil(s) with your affirmations. Then take inventory of your emotions throughout the different situations you encounter daily, weekly, and/or monthly.
- Do daily tapping exercises.
- Exercise three or more times per week.
- Get a nutrition and wellness checkup.
- Reassess your dietary needs (you can never learn enough about health and wellness).
- See a therapist or counselor to help with insight and techniques for changes tailored to your needs.
- Find a support group if you need people to talk to.
- See a chiropractor if your body is feeling out of alignment. As you've learned throughout this book, an unbalanced body can create an unbalanced mind. The information I provide should help you realize when you're mind/body aren't in sync.

Like with any exercise program, you should do as many of the exercises in this book as often as possible until you're comfortable doing them. Then keep doing them as practice makes perfect!

They'll become easier over time, and before you know it you'll begin to feel better. But they only work if you're committed to your well-being (ergo, believe and faith) by staying on task with what you need to do every single day.

## Rising to a Higher Level of Awareness

Use your imagination for a moment to dream (in present tense) what it feels like to wake up energized and looking forward to your day. Imagine what it feels like to be free from headaches, fatigue, or depression. Then Imagine what it feels like to be the person you've longed to be.

Take a moment to reflect on the issues you're struggling with that are preventing you from achieving them. Then rate them on a scale from 0 to 10 (0 being the worst, and 0 not at all). The following are a few examples, so add your own if they're missing:

_____ not loving yourself
_____ lacking self-confidence
_____ feeling isolated
_____ emotional turmoil
_____ easily irritated
_____ anger
_____ rage
_____ depression
_____ poor diet
_____ lack of exercise
_____ nightmares or night terrors
_____ flashbacks
_____ avoidance of places, things, smells, people, etc.
_____ paranoia
_____ anxiety
_____ despair
_____ regret
_____ humiliation
_____ blame
_____ _____ (something not listed)

How long have you had one or more of these symptoms?

_____

In the past, have people tried to get you help and you refused?
_____ Yes _____ No

If you refused help, what were your reasons?

_____
_____
_____

Can you think back to a time where you felt confident in yourself?
_____ Yes _____ No

If yes, why did you feel that way?

_____
_____
_____

What helped you to feel confident?

_____
_____
_____

How can you apply that to your situation to regain your confidence?

_____
_____
_____

# Exercise:
## Visualizing Your Changes

Close your eyes. Cross your arms over your chest, and places your hands on your shoulders. Alternate tapping on your shoulder muscles while visualizing yourself overcoming your present feelings and emotions.

Then write down how the situation began to shift.

_____
_____
_____

Now I want you to see yourself making these changes. On a scale of 0 to 10 (10 being "I will overcome these issues"), what number would your rate the current issue? _____

If you couldn't make the transition from a negative to positive mental state of mind, what stopped you?

_____
_____
_____

Repeat this exercise as many times as you need with different emotions and/or states of mind you're dealing with.

If you get stuck in negativity, use frankincense with the following affirmation: *"I choose to release all trauma that no longer serves me. I choose peace."* As you repeat this, allow yourself to transition to a calm, still place in your mind described earlier.

## How the Lack of Energy (Electricity) Can Affect Your Health

The three major natural life forces essential to your body's survival are electricity, water, and oxygen. If your body goes very long without any of these, the result can be very detrimental to your health.

During his research, Dr. Robert Becker (an orthopedic surgeon at SUNY Upstate working for the Veterans Administration) began to understand how electricity promoted healing and well-being (SEE: *The Body Electric: Electromagnetism and the Foundation of Life*). Unfortunately, he was before his time, or before society could adjust to the paradigm shift he was presenting.

Many people have never thought of their body as having electricity or internal "voltage." Just as your car or house uses electricity, your body does as well. To bring vitality into your body, you need your internal "batteries" to function properly.

### Electricity 101A

Your body has one of the most complex electrical systems on the planet. Every day I'm amazed at what scientists are learning about the body's electrical system.

Essential oils allow the body to support electrical activity. If your electrical system isn't functioning as well as it should be, a harmonic state of balance will be difficult to achieve. Therefore, an imbalanced electrical system is a sign that you're experiencing less than optimal health.

In early science classes in school, you probably learned about protons, electrons, and neutrons that assist the body in key functions. For example, a loss in electricity or electrons can result in decreased essential oxygen in your body. This will create a chain reaction, much like tossing a large rock into a lake and the ripples affect the entire lake.

The electrical signals in your brain help govern your circadian rhythms (your "internal body clock"). These are your natural rhythms your body goes through during a 24-hour period to regulate the release of hormones, metabolic rate, body temperature, and many other activities in your body.

If your circadian rhythms become out of balance, it can be difficult to be in sync with the rise and fall of the sun. For example, at night your brain creates melatonin that tells your body it's time to shift into a state of *theta* where you're not awake but not asleep.

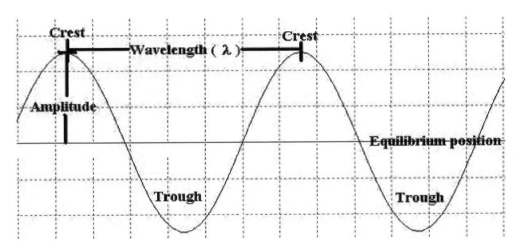

This diagram illustrating the scientific terms of the brain's electrical activity is used only for educational purposes.

The *delta* state will follow as you begin to grow tired. *Delta* – the main frequency utilized while you're asleep – is the brain wave frequency of 1 to 4 cycles per second. Versus *beta* – the main frequency of being awake and alert – that's an average of 16 cycles per second.

For those in the scientific world, delta has a much higher amplitude with a wider trough (slow activity). Whereas beta has a lower amplitude and a narrower trough, which allows for more cycles per second and a higher brain frequency. So with anxiety issues, faster brain states such as beta can be a problem. With depression, slower states such as delta and theta can also be an issue.

The goal is to be able to shift into the appropriate frequency whenever you need to. For example, as the day is winding down around 7:00 p.m. or so, your theta frequency causes you to be less alert and puts you in the delta mode of sleep.

Being in a beta state throughout the day is an indicator of sympathetic lock because your body isn't allowed to relax or be calm. Thus, your mind will often be running or racing which can be difficult to control.

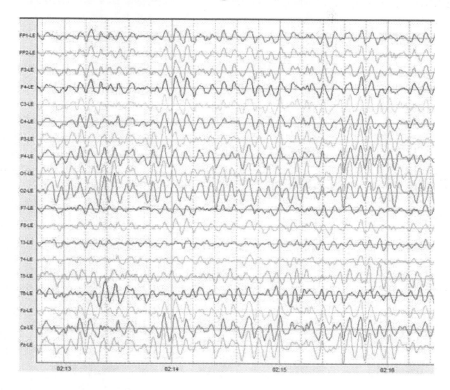

The above image taken of the brain's electroencephalogram
or EEG on the International 10-20 locations is being used only for
educational purposes. This is the raw EEG
utilized through Neuroguide.

The image shows that not all of the lines are the same. All you need to understand from this example is their brain wasn't in balance as some parts were going faster than others.

## How Does Your Brain Work?

Not everyone can be an Albert Einstein. But most everyone wants their brain to work as good as it possibly can.

There are many different aspects that go into long-lasting brain health. For good brain health you want healthy, positive habits such as exercise, eating right, wholesome friendships, and strong spiritual beliefs.

The before-and-after images on the chart below are from an individual diagnosed with PTSD by using standardized testing measures and clinical observation. I'm sharing them with you to give you a greater understanding of neuroplasticity and possibilities for healing (meaning, your brain can change, and you don't have to be permanently stuck with your symptoms).

Here's a quick run-through of the chart's terms for people interested in the science behind  brain mapping:

- **Power** represents the microvolts square/hertz, which tells you the power of different locations of the brain. Both absolute and relative power play a role in providing significant information to a clinician.

  The absolute power ratio is different from the relative power ratio in that absolute power doesn't take into account an individual's facts such as skull thickness, skin differences, etc.

- **Asymmetry** is the amplitude, or the rise and fall, of the frequencies in different brain areas. You don't want the amplitude to be so high that your mind becomes foggy (higher equals slower frequencies), or so low that your mind thinks too fast. There are times to think, and times to sleep. So your brain's ability to shift between states is very important.

- **Coherence** tells you the the difference between the brain's left and right hemispheres, and how they communicate together. You don't want the brain to communicate too much between the hemispheres, as it would be like your siblings knowing all about your married life. That's way too much information!

Though it's best to not see lines of any color in the asymmetry or coherence, the green ranges in the power measures demonstrate normal brain connectivity.

Outside these ranges would indicate a measure outside the normative range. A good place to be is in the normative range where the majority of the world's population lies. Two standard deviations out would indicate a potential clinical issue.

The red lines indicate high brain connectivity, whereas the blue lines indicate slow brain connectivity. In the power ranges, the blue and red are outside the norm, whereas the green is within the standard normative range. All of which refers to frequency (delta, theta, alpha, beta, high beta, and gamma respectively).

Therefore, the heads themselves represent delta 1-4 hertz, theta 4-8 hertz, and alpha 8-12 hertz.

*(The words above the heads and the color chart refer to range.)*

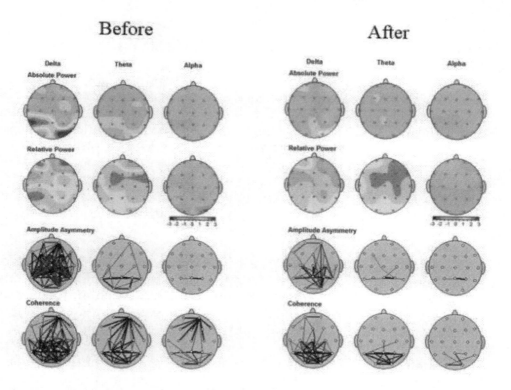

Disclaimer: WPHC and our affliates can't verify if every person will or won't obtain these same kinds of results and for how long.
Since theraputic outcomes differ from person to person,
the images above are only used for educational purposes. These images were captured by Ryan via Brain Master Discovery hardware, and processed through a Neuroguide normative database.

Looking at the two absolute power ratios of the different heads, you can see that there are differences in colors between the before and after images. In the absolute power ratio, the after set of images has much more green, which is the average or norm.

The red and blue lines are fast and slow relationships. Therefore, in the before image you can see that the prefrontal cortex sites (Fp1, Fp2, F7, F8, and Fz related to the 10 to 20 international sites) on the top of the head are different between the before and after images.

The after absolute power images in the spectrum analysis no longer show any red, which indicates that the individual was able to return to a normal standard deviation pattern. Simply put, this would help illustrate how essential oils can help support the brain, or a better level of homeostasis. The conclusion is this is a positive modality that appears to be beneficial for the individual.

## Methods to Determine Brain Trauma

*(This section provides basic beneficial information for individuals suffering from PTSD and extreme trauma.)*

You might wonder if there are ways to change what's occuring in your brain. My answer would be yes, as I firmly believe the physical brain (versus the mind) can be altered.

My colleagues have demonstrated that changes in different regions of the brain can occur in as little as 20 minutes after neurofeedback training.

The article "Surface and LORETA Neurofeedback in the Treatment of Post-Traumatic Stress Disorder and Mild Traumatic Brain Injury" by Drs. Dale Foster and Thatcher discusses the research outcomes of individuals with PTSD and mild brain injuries. These studies validate the different modalities used to support the field of neuroplasticity.

Another article "Z-score LORETA Neurofeedback As a Potential Therapy for Depression/Anxiety and Cognitive Dysfunction" by J. L. Koberda discusses potential outcomes with brain training for people struggling with such issues. (URLs for both articles in References)

An EEG (electroencephalography) detects brain wave activity and functioning, whereas an MRI (Magnetic Resonance Imaging) uses magnets and radio waves on a part of the body being tested. Though an MRI is somewhat different from an EEG, both demonstrate different areas of concern for individuals struggling with trauma or other mental health conditions.

Psychiatrist Dr. Daniel Amen developed the SPECT (Single Photon Emission Computed Tomography) that measure the brain's blood flow and activity.

He's written several books that discuss his treatment model that includes the key role of the limbic system (or the "deep limbic" system as he calls it, a term he uses to illustrate the brain's temporal lobes and the cingulate gyrus).

Deep within the brain are the deep temporal lobes (the amygdala, hippocampus and anterior thalamic nuclei) that are about the size of a walnut.

Amen states the deep limbic system is responsible for *"Setting the emotional tone of the mind, filters external events through internal states, tag events as internally important, stores highly charged emotional memories, modulates motivation, controls appetite and sleep cycles, promotes bonding, directly processes the sense of smell, modulates libido."* (Amen, *Change Your Brain, Change Your Life*, 2015).

Dr. Amen also states that individuals diagnosed with PTSD are seen with a "diamond shape pattern from the prefrontal cortex, basal ganglia, and limbic system," or the different areas of the brain that play into this traumatic condition.

As I analyze Neurofeedback Training (NFT) brain maps, I'm often concerned about the hypothalamus-pituitary-adrenal axis (HPA), the area of the brain that can affect stress response, fight-or-flight issues, and emotional irregularity.

In his book, *Getting Started With Neurofeedback*, John Demos states, "Davidson and Irwin (1999) reported a unique connection between the visual cortex, the amygdala, and PTSD." During their study of how the intensity of fear relates to brain function, they observed an increased blood flow to the left amygdala.

Demos discusses other research that arrived at the same conclusion about the relationship between these areas of the brain and PTSD. Individuals subjected to NFT have reported positive gains in these areas of the brain. The research showed how the brain receives information, and the fastest ways to affect the amygdala (interestingly, the sense of smell is the only one that goes through one synapse to the brain):

*"[The brain's] 100 billion or so nerve cells, which constitute the brain's hardware, are able to store more information than all of the libraries in the world combined. Each of these nerve cells (neurons) is in turn composed of three basic elements. The nucleus of the cell body (soma) constitutes a miniature brain within a larger brain. It is the soma that 'decides' to transmit a message (an electrical impulse) from one nerve cell to the next, that is, to 'fire.'*

*Or the soma may decide to ignore the message, that is, to 'not fire.' This is the only decision the soma needs to make, but it needs to make that decision very quickly.*

*For example, you don't want to wait 5 minutes to remove the hand you unknowingly placed on the hot stove whole the soma takes its time deciding to transmit the message to the next neuron and ultimately on to the brain.*

*Like a computer, the soma is a 'fast idiot.' It has to make one of only two possible decisions, that is, to fire or not to fire.*

*Connected to the soma is a long fiber, the axon, through which the message must travel on it way to the next neuron. The message is transferred from one of the many branches at the end of the axon of the sending neuron to one of a number of branches on the receiving cell. These branches on the receiving cell are called dendrites; each neuron may have up to 10,000 dendrites.*

*If we consider the possibilities of interaction among the 100 billion neurons found in the human brain with 10,000 dendrites per neuron, we have the possibility of quadrillions of connection-different ways to send messages to different 'receivers,' with different results. Clearly, as we have said, the brain is the most complex entity in this universe."* (Milkman and Sunderwith, *Cravings for Ecstasy and Natural Highs*, 2010)

Understanding neuronal action at its most basic level shows how information in the brain is transferred. The brain communicates with itself and the rest of the body through different frequencies, which in turn can alter an individual's moods:

*"Indeed, the brain is a giant pharmaceutical factory constantly manufacturing chemicals that result in moods such as fear, anger, shame, despair, joy, depression, mania, and many other mood to which the human species is subjected."* (Milkman and Sunderwith, 2010)

Neurochemicals also play an important part during the information transmission process. For example:

*"Blum (1991) has proposed a model for reward (pleasure) involving the interaction of several neurotransmitters with the various parts of the limbic system that composes the reward center. The release of dopamine into the nucleus accumbens, an important reward site, plays a major role in medicating our moods.*

*Although there are other reward sites in the limbic system, for simplicity we will limit our discussion to the action of dopamine on the nucleus accumbens.*

*In Blum's model, which he calls the reward cascade, feelings of well-being, as well as the absence of cravings and anxiety, depend on an adequate supply of dopamine flowing into the nucleus accumbens. Dopamine mediates the reward properties of both natural and drug-induced pleasures."* (Carelli, *The Nucleus Accumbens and Reward,* 2001)

*In humans, any imbalance that would lead to a deficit of dopamine would produce anxiety and cravings for substances (alcohol, cocaine, heroin, amphetamine, etc.) or activities (e.g. gambling, crime, promiscuous sex, hang gliding) that would temporarily restore this deficit."* (Milkman and Sunderwith, 2010)

Neurochemicals also play a very important role in how you feel and behave. Pharmaceutical drugs attempt to assist the body in the regulation of such chemicals. The problem I see with that is if your body can make dopamine – but due to a stimulus or stressor is unable to properly regulate it – it's essential to understand why the natural process no longer works properly.

In other words, are you paying attention to your body's signals about the issues it's facing? This information can be determined via blood work, hair and energetic analysis, and many other methods that can help you learn about how your body functions.

Remember, you can only benefit from a plan that you believe will help. So choosing a practitioner who has the correct credentials will increase your faith in the plan's ability to work.

## Your Body Electric!

One way to look at your body's energy activity is with a gas discharge visualization camera (GDV). It's believed that Semyon Kirlian accidentally discovered a high voltage corona field (aura of color) on a leaf (https://en.wikipedia.org/wiki/Kirlian_photography). Although the photography method has been altered over the years, the foundation of the science is still active today.

Another source of measuring your body's voltage is with a voltage meter since voltage can be measured by the body's wiring system.

*"The body has two wiring systems that carry voltage to each organ. One wiring system is called the Perineural Nervous System, and is actually a sheath around each nerve. The other is the acupuncture system, and is actually the fascial planes of the body. Thus we commonly use an ohmmeter to measure and then convert that to voltage."* (Tennant, 2013)

A negative attitude decreases the flow of electricity and number of electrons throughout your body. The lower the number of electrons, the more difficult it is for your body to heal, thus achieving lower ATP and oxygen levels. Therefore, this will work best when thinking about something positive or enjoyable.

*"Our thoughts and emotions combine to form vibrations – frequencies – our 'line of resistance'. Our thoughts, mingled with either love or fear, will create our experiences that will then manifest in our lives physically, mentally, and spiritually, either as health or disease."* ~Dr. Carey Reams

Dr. Bruce Lipton, a premier scientist who's studied the principles of quantum physics, teaches that your vibrations can affect every molecule you come into contact with. Therefore, you are much more than just your genetics and/or DNA.

For many years scientists have used MRIs and other testing methods to observe genes to determine what genes cause what problems. The information that's been found in people's genes is very important, as it can provide a foundation of why some people struggle with certain issues more than others.

Over time stress will expose any weakness in your genes. This is very important to understand as gene weakness, in spite of a healthy lifestyle, might never manifest an issue.

I'm confident that quantum physics and other scientific methods can teach people a great deal about their personal beliefs. For instance, Dr. Masaru Emoto (a certified doctor of alternative medicine) and his staff took photographs of different kinds of frozen water, hoping to see different kinds of crystal formations:

*"At first, we strenuously observed crystals of tap water, river water, and lake water. From the tap water we could not get any beautiful crystals. We could not get any beautiful ones from rivers and lakes near big cities, either. However, from the water from rivers and lakes where water is kept pristine from development, we could observe beautiful crystals with each one having its own uniqueness.*

*The observation was done in various ways: Observe the crystal of frozen water after showing letters to water. Showing pictures to water. Playing music to water. Praying to water.*

*In all of these experiments, distilled water for hospital usage produced by the same company was used. Since it is distilled twice, it can be said that it is pure water.*

*The result was that we always observed beautiful crystals after giving good words, playing good music, and showing, playing, or offering pure prayer to water."* (You can either search for his work on the Internet to find different images of his work. Or go to his website listed in References.)

Dr. Emoto conducted these experiments to illustrate the impact of good/bad frequency on water. In essence, his resulting photographs show that water has memory. Therefore, praying over and/or blessing your words with positive thoughts will be absorbed by and affect your body.

His photographic results (that can be found in his astounding series of books, *Messages from Water*) are very impressive. They're a clear indication that your thoughts and beliefs can have a huge impact on your life.

Old, negative patterns and habits can be hard to detect. Once you begin to alter your vibrations, you'll notice them more by following these steps:

1. Be patient with yourself during the learning curve.
2. Fully experience your emotions, as it can be an amazing source of self-discovery.
3. Focus on why you feel the way you do.
4. Are there past experiences that still affect you in the present? To paraphrase Alcoholics Anonymous' (AA) fourth step: "Make a searching moral and fearless inventory of yourself." (From the Alcoholics Anonymous Big Book).

Emotions create an unseen magnet field, thus creating a resonance or a dissonance in your body. The song, *Good Vibrations*, by the iconic American band, the Beach Boys, is a great way to understand emotional vibrations.

*I love the colorful clothes she wears,*
*And the way the sunlight plays upon her hair.*
*I hear the sound of a gentle word*
*On the wind that lifts her perfume through the air.*
*I'm picking up good vibrations.*
*She's giving me excitations.*
*Good bop bop, good vibrations.*
*Bop bop, excitations.*
*Good, good, good, good vibrations.*

When you're around someone for the first time, you might get a certain feeling about them. What you're sensing is their frequency or vibration. Some people have a very positive vibration, and you want to be around them all the time. Whereas others give off a negative vibration, much like touching an electrical fence that warns you there's danger and you should stay away.

You might have seen someone dancing by themselves during a worship service or at a concert in a very beautful, creative way. The people watching them might think they're crazy, while others will enjoy it, and some will even join in.

Which brings to mind a professor at Hardin Simmons University (whom I'll always remember) who loved to dance during a worship service at his church where he was a member.

He'd been struggling with how he felt about the way people saw him and his new behavior. But the genuine excitement, vibrations and emotions he felt moved him past his fear of acceptance into pure joy and elation. He no longer worried about what people thought of him because the celebration of dance brought his spirit closer to God.

If your thoughts are positive, and you're passionate about your life, then the resonance within your body will be much stronger. Plus, you'll be able to obtain those higher calibrated emotional states I mentioned earlier.

On the other hand, if you're negative about your life, your magnet field will be weaker. Removing negative emotional magnetic fields will bring forth a stronger state in your body.

*In other words, your thoughts can positively or affect your body's well-being.*

# Exercise:
## "Oiling" Your Electromagnetic Centers

Essential oils can help increase your body's electrical activity. Some people might have a very unique experience the first time they put an oil on their body.

Some individuals report they immediately taste the oil as if it were in their mouth, or smell it as if it were right below their nostrils. While others say they can't feel any difference.

These kinds of results are accomplished in several ways:

- One way is to put oil on all electromagnetic centers to keep them in balance while clearing negative emotions. Some people refer to these areas as *chakras*, whereas I prefer to call them *electromagnetic centers*.

Although there are numerous electromagnetic centers, I prefer to use seven as it aligns with numerous teachings of the Jewish culture. The traditional menorah aligns with all seven centers of the body (seven pipes supplying oil to seven lamps, etc.). "Those seven are the eyes of the Lord, ranging over the whole earth." (Zachariah 4:1-10, Tanakh)

The image below shows the misalignment of electromagnetic centers before the person utilized tapping, meditation and oils. However, if you line them up in the center of the image, you can see where the oils should go.

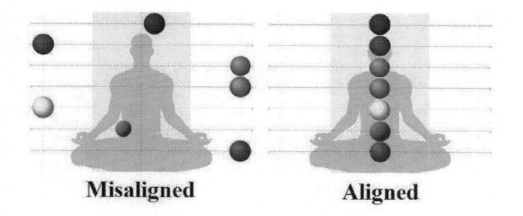

**Misaligned**              **Aligned**

Because the colored circles were centered and in alignment, the person reported feeling calm and peaceful after applying the oils.

- Or you can put an oil like vetiver on one or more electromagnetic centers 3 or 4 times per day. Or as often as you want, especially if you're trying to clear negative emotions in numerous places.

Your hands and feet have reflex points, so applying oils to them are a great way to get the maximum benefits (you can Google reflex charts on the Internet to find the right locations to apply the oils).

If you're new to using essential oils, they can be combined or used individually. Oftentimes I'll blend them together for ease of application and to save time. You might begin with lemon, lavender, frankincense, cedarwood, sage, vetiver, or an oil of your choice.

Place the oil(s) in the well of your hand, stir clockwise three or four times, then apply the oil from the bottom of your chin down to just above the belt line.

Doing this can help decrease negative emotions, lower your pulse rate, and keep the parasympathetic engaged (out of fight-or-flight). Over time, this will become much easier to sense and hold on to.

## Tuning Forks and The Frequencies of Stored Emotions

The entire world is an "ocean of motion." Even Mother Nature illustrates her powerful energy in storms, tornados, hurricanes and other forms of environmental conditions.

Isaac Newton's Theory of Motion states that everything is either stationary, or keeps on going until you give it a push.

Your entire body (including your organs) vibrate at certain rates, which are referenced as *hertz* in the frequencies of the harmonics with sound. (Musical notes are very useful, as the harmonics in hertz can be converted for anything.)

Not only have I used tuning forks to tune a musical instrument, I've used them with every client dealing with an emotional release because they're tuned to frequencies or notes, much like music.

As a basic rule of thumb, the forks can be held over the body about six inches or so as they vibrate. Or placed directly over the organ, or on the organ's meridian line.

*The Essential Oil Desk References* shows which oils can be used for general support of the organ's system. The location of the oil can either be on your feet, your back, or over the organ.

Some people sense many different sensations as the oils are placed in different locations. But those teachings are more technical, and beyond the scope of this basic workbook.

Listed below are the musical notes and frequencies of ancient understanding:

| Organ | Frequency/ Note |
|---|---|
| Adrenals | 492.8 (E b) |
| Bladder | 352 (F) |
| Brain | 315.8 (E b) |
| Colon | 176 (F) |
| Gall Bladder | 164.3 (E) |
| Pancreas | 117.3 (C #) |
| Lungs | 220 (A) |
| Stomach | 110 (A) |
| Liver | 317.83 (E b) |
| Intestines | 281 (C#) |
| Bone | 418 (A b) |
| Muscles | 324 (E) |

SEE: http://greatdreams.com/hertz.htm

## How to Put All of This Together

The usage of tuning forks pulls many complex scientific methods together. (Many companies offer a variety of forks and methods in which you can use them. Plus there are many Essential Oil Desk References available online.)

| Organs | Associate Emotion |
|---|---|
| Liver | Anger |
| Kidney-Bladder | Fear, shame, guilt, broken will |
| Spleen-Stomach | Anxiety, broken power, low self-worth |
| Heart-Small Intestine | Loneliness, humiliation, abandonment, insecurity |
| Lung-Large Intestine | Grief |
| Sympathetic- Parasympathetic | Anxiety |

From: Tennant, *Healing is Voltage*

To support the liver, and emotions related to this organ, I'd use an E-flat note a tuning fork is tuned to. Then apply an essential oil over the liver that would support that organ, such as juniper or ledum. This method would also help deal with emotions of anger.

(Though I haven't been trained in her methods, this is one reason why the Vibrational Raindrop Method created by Dr. Christi Bonds-Garrett, M.D. is so powerful. For further information, see drbondsgarrett.com.)

The above method uses more advanced skills, which can be applied to the individual in very unique ways. I'm only mentioning it to show you there's a great deal that can be discussed. But this workbook was purely written as an introduction to essential oil uses, and the different energy methods in which they can be used.

## Listen to Your Body

Emotions can be both conscious or unconscious. One isn't more powerful than the other, but most people's emotions are subconscious. Subconscious thoughts can send you into fight-or-flight just as fast as your conscious thoughts.

Emotions can exist in physical locations (known as "blocks" where emotions affect an organ's function). From Dr. Tennant's *Healing is Voltage*, below are examples of emotions and their physical locations to help you understand what your body is trying to tell you:

Louise Hays's iconic book, *Heal Your Body*, lists the organs then the negative feeling, and the positive affirmation that goes with it. (Too many to list here, they can also be found at the Alchemy of Healing Website: http://alchemyofhealing.com/causes-of-symptoms-according-to-louise-hay/).

Freeing your body's energy allows a stronger sense of balance to be obtained. This is a great way to think about how all organs have a frequency as well as emotions, and how emotions can become stored in your body (a concept not taught in traditional high-level American educational institutions).

## Exercise:
## Balancing Your Electrical Currents

If you want to try to feel your body's energy, placing a drop of an oil like frankincense on one wrist, then rubbing both wrists together, will help open your body's electrical flow.

I began teaching people how to do this after I learned a technique at the Center for Aromatherapy Research and Education where someone helps you balance your electrical activity.

I don't always have someone available to help me with my tasks in the office. So one day while praying and mediating, the Lord enlightened me with this approach which I now use with myself and my clients.

In the beginning you might not feel much, or you might question if you're doing it right. It can take up to three or four minutes, and in some cases even longer, to feel a subtle pulse or a tingling feeling. If your heart rate is over 95 beats per minute, it might take even longer. Also, the more blocks you have in your energy circuits, the longer it will take.

The longer you do this, the quicker and easier it will become. Plus, increasing your senses allows you to be more in the present moment with this activity.

- Close your eyes.
- Focus on your breathing and how you're feeling.
- Count to 4 as you inhale, then to 6 as you exhale. Your breath rate will help the coherence of the information being sent between the brain and the body, which will then be generated much quicker to your entire body.

For people with more chronic issues, it might take up to five minutes or longer.

Just like cooking in the kitchen, you want to keep your body's electrical circuitry working well so it can "keep cooking" internally. Be patient, practice often, and you'll eventually become in tune with your body's energy (electricity) where you'll feel a subtle vibration or a slight pulse.

Think back to what you were feeling before you began the exercise. On a scale of 0 to 10 (0 being low stress to 10 being high stress), what do you think your stress level was? _____

What did you experience after doing this exercise?

_____
_____
_____

How do you feel now emotionally, mentally and physically compared to how you felt before?

_____
_____
_____

Now that you learned some basic techniques to determine your emotional states and energy (or lack thereof), this next chapter will teach you how to remove any emotional blocks preventing your healing.

# Energetically Removing
# Emotional Blocks

While studying many different energetic approaches, such as those listed above and others, I often ask the Lord how to use them for myself. Other people's approaches don't always match my style, so that's where I use my creativity and inspiration (and you can as well).

*The Emotion Code* by Dr. Bradley Nelson teaches people how to release limiting emotions. Because I already knew about tapping, and how the governing lines of the body work energetically, I really didn't need to learn about magnets.

But since I understand the frequency and energy of essential oils, I decided to create my own approach based on a combination of affirmations, tapping and Dr. Nelson's findings. (I encourage you to study his work as he's a very gifted holistic physician.)

Remember, your heart has an electromagnetic field stronger than any other field in your body. When you introduce something as powerful as an essential oil into this field, your body feels it. So combining this method with your intent is all you need to make the shift in your consciousness.

The goal in my approach is to remove emotional, generational, heart and birth blocks. For this process I use vetiver and/or frankincense essential oils. I specifically use them because they always give the best results. (However, if you feel you'd benefit more from different oils, by all means feel free to try them.)

I don't put the oils directly on the person's body to remove emotions. Instead, I hold the bottle about an inch or so above the person's body while "tracing" an imaginary line from the belt line on the front of their body to the belt line on the back of their body (see image below). The closer to the person's body I can get, the better. But I'm very careful to respect their boundaries.

Once I reach their brow line, I place my left index fingertip on the middle of their forehead. Then with my right hand I gently "karate chop" the back of their head. (I do the tapping after I first run the bottle over their body.)

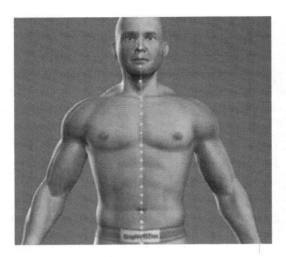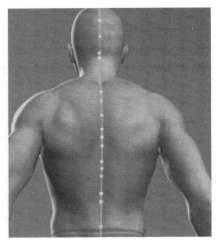

These images were taken via the app Easy Acupuncture.
The full version is available on iTunes or Google Play.

For blocks other than generational issues, the bottle needs to be "floated" over the body three or more times. Feel free to do more, but a minimum of three passes works well. Generational blocks take more energy to remove, so the bottle must float over the body ten or more times.

While doing this exercise, you might notice a shift in your emotions. Most people feel peaceful and calm. I've had some people cry, some laugh, and some not feel a thing. But they all report the numerous different emotions they felt during and after their body work.

Because this is a very powerful method, I only use it only when the body is willing. So I first use kinesiology to determine their needs. In most cases people can only remove about three to six blocks during each session or per day. I encourage you to not do more than your body can handle as it can create a state of imbalance.

You might ask what a block is, and which blocks need to be released. The unconscious brain stores blocks of emotions in any organ or layer of an individual's being throughout their body. Just like with the Biowell images, seeing the gasses your body emits is a great way to determine the blocks needing to be dealt with.

You can also refer back to the earlier section, "Listen to Your Body" that lists different emotions. Any of those emotion(s) you're struggling with can be released.

Almost every person I've worked with came in with some form of birth trauma. People who didn't experience much trauma, or at all, typically were delivered naturally during a water birth, or in a natural environment such as a prearranged home birth.

If you don't know the specifics around your birth, try to find out what they were (easy, difficult, traumatic, etc.). Then try to release the trauma during one of these sessions. For example, when I was born I had a hematoma (a collection of blood outside a blood vessel) on my head. Because that was a traumatic circumstance, I've used muscle testing and kinesiology to determine the emotions and the origins of the issue.

I also had other issues resulting from my parents' relationship which needed to be released. It took many sessions over a period of time to shed the different layers of trauma.

It's best if someone can help you during this process, as doing it by yourself can be very tricky. If you can't find someone to assist you, just do your best. Or you can visit churches or organizations in your community to create a support system.

*NOTE: If you want to learn more about muscle testing, I have information that teaches you how to do it correctly. You can contact me via my email address at the end of the book to find out how to purchase the downloadable document.*

*Also, if you want to learn more about how to release "emotionally-charged events from your past that can still be haunting you in the form of 'trapped emotions'," you can read* The Emotion Code *by Dr. Nelson, then use the method I mentioned above.*

## Learning to Forgive

I'd like to conclude my workbook with an example of forgiveness. Forgiveness mostly affects the prefrontal cortex, or the front part of your brain. As you struggle with forgiveness, this part of the brain becomes overactive, which causes a chain reaction in your body's chemistry and electrical activity.

The resulting behaviors are issues with impulse control and executive functions this part of the brain does. If this occurs, the electrical activity of this area needs to be corrected.

Correcting this area will involve your nutritional needs, your thoughts, your emotions, your chemistry, your electricity and your habits.

# Exercise:
## Assessing Your Forgiveness

*"We cannot embrace God's forgiveness if we are so busy clinging to past wounds and nursing old grudges."*
~T.D. Jakes

Harboring ill feelings can create a hardened heart. They can build a high wall that will prevent you from connecting positively with others.

Once you've identified what emotions are associated with your trauma, the next step is forgiveness.

Has anything prevented you from forgiving yourself or others?
_____ Yes _____ No.

If yes, please explain why:

_____

_____

_____

On a scale of 1 to 10 (10 being the best), how are you doing with forgiveness? _____

What steps can you take to release bad feelings and begin to forgive (this includes yourself)?

_____

_____

_____

Becoming more in touch with your feelings can be frightening and intimidating. But you can always return to this book to remind you that ***you are not alone!***

All roads are intended to lead to the same destination. So based on what you've learned in this book, you now have many to choose from to begin your journey to wellness.

# PART III

# BONUS CHAPTER
# SAMPLE TIPS, TOOLS AND RECIPES

*WARNING: Be careful not to get the oils (especially the hot oils) near your eyes as they can cause an uncomfortable burning sensation. If you do, quickly rub a small amount of carrier oil like olive or coconut oil around your eyes for immediate relief. Never splash water on your eyes as water will open your pores and cause more discomfort. Then gently dab your eyes with a towel. Repeat if necessary. Don't use eye drops as they can cause the oil to burn even hotter.*

*The following are just some simple basics, and not meant to be a comprehensive guide. There are many resources on the Internet, or in bookstores – and even on our Facebook pages and websites – that provide additional information. This is just a "teaser" to let you know how many practical uses there are for essential oils!*

Earlier you were given a comprehensive list of the most common essential oils used in aromatherapy. Now we're going to give you some practical applications for some of the most common issues people use them for. (In his workbook, Ryan discusses how they can be used to overcome many kinds of traumas.)

Remember to always keep your essential oils handy, as you never know when you need them!

(Some of the following information and recipes, which will be noted as such, were generously provided by the Sapp's daughters, Abby and Paige.)

## Topical and Internal Uses for Essential Oils

*Seasonal Changes in the Air: (Pollen Punch-Out from Abby)*

Not only does this work great for our dog, Jake, but for Mom's reactions due to the dog.

4 drops of lemongrass
4 drops of tea tree
4 drops of rosemary
4 drops of citronella
8 drops of thyme

Add everything to 8 ounces of filtered or distilled water in a glass spray bottle, then shake well. You can adjust the amount of drops of essential oils based on the size of the bottle.

*Anxiousness:*

1 to 2 drops each of frankincense and lavender oils

Rub the oils on your pulse points to help you become relaxed, calm and grounded. The oils can be applied multiple times per day until you feel better.

*Bad Breath (from Abby)*

I call this the "Death Breath Spray."

1 drop of spearmint essential oil
1 drop of peppermint essential oil
Small glass spray bottle (we got our tiny inexpensive spray bottles from myoilgear.com).

Pour mouthwash of your choice (we recommend natural and organic without toxic chemicals) into the spray bottle. Then add the drops of oil. Shake to mix. The oils help the mouthwash last longer, and increases its benefit by several times.

*Bee Stings:*

Hundreds of thousands, if not millions, of people are allergic to bee stings. Always keep your EpiPen handy, especially during hot or smoky weather as that angers bees. This isn't meant to replace the EpiPen that contains epinephrine to aid in anaphylactic shock, respiratory shutdowns, or severe skin/breathing reactions. But it will help bring relief to your skin after you've been stung. It can also work on mosquito and other bug bites as well.

The following oils can relieve the agitation, swelling, stinging and itchiness:

chamomile
lavender
peppermint
tansy
wintergreen

Wasps and hornets don't leave a stinger that contain venom behind, but bees do. If you're stung by a bee, you can use a credit card to swipe it from your skin, or place tobacco or mud on the sting. Add water to make a paste, then apply it to the sting area. The stinger will be drawn out as the paste dries.

Once the stinger has been removed, apply 1 to 2 drops directly to the area every15 minutes for the first hour. Then the oils can be applied multiple times per day until the redness and swelling subside. You can also apply a cold compress on the area to reduce swelling.

Note:  Peppermint oil seems to repel bees. So if you're in an area that has bees, you can apply peppermint to your clothing and skin to keep them away.

WARNING: Since peppermint is a hot oil, you might want to first apply a carrier oil to your skin.

*Breathing Issues:*

Place 1 to 2 drops of peppermint oil in the palm of your hand. Rub your hands together, then place both palms in front of your face without touching it. Slowly inhale then exhale for several minutes at a time. This process is commonly used after dealing with seasonal changes and pollens in the air.

*Chapped Lips (from Paige):*

Here's the recipe for my Mint Chocolate Lip Balm:

5 Tablespoons coconut oil
3 Tablespoons beeswax
12 drops peppermint essential oil (you can use other oils such as lavender, orange, lemon, citrus fresh, lime, etc., to change the scent and flavor. You can even add a little organic vanilla.)
1/8 to 1/4 teaspoon cocoa powder

Put the coconut oil and beeswax in a microwave safe measuring cup. Microwave until melted (be watchful as it doesn't take long. Start at 10-15 second intervals. Keep going until the wax is melted.) If you don't want to use a microwave, put the coconut oil and beeswax in a saucepan over low heat until they're melted.

Take out the cup (or remove the pan from the stove) and stir well. Then add your essential oil of choice, cocoa powder, and stir well. Pour the liquid into containers (I use containers about the size of a quarter that have screw-on lids. But feel free to experiment with different ways to store your lip balm.)

Your lips will feel and smell FUN-omen-OIL!

*Circulation:*

This wonderful blended oil you can massage into weary muscles and aching joints can be created by blending together the following essential oils:

eucalyptus
juniper
lemongrass
marjoram
peppermint
thyme
vetiver
wintergreen

...with a carrier oil such as:

almond oil
coconut oil (fractionated)
grape seed oil
olive oil
or wheat germ oil

Put the blend and carrier oil in a small glass spray bottle you can use at home, at work, or while traveling to ease "tired bum" syndrome or circulation to enliven your body and your spirits. You can use a small Mason jar (about 1 cup size) with a lid to keep your blend secure if it tips over.

*Cramps:*

Some of the best oils for any type of cramping is peppermint and wintergreen. These are "hot" oils, so use them with a carrier oil such as coconut or olive.

First put in about 3 to 4 tablespoons of the carrier oil into a cup-size Mason jar with a lid. Then add about 10 drops of peppermint and wintergreen oils.

Tighten the lid, then shake it together. Keep your new blend in a cool environment like your home. Keep it handy to use as often as needed!

*Fever Blisters:*

A great way to deal with fever blisters is to use a small bottle that can hold 2 to 3 teaspoons of liquid.

Drop 20 to 25 each of the following essential oils into the bottle:

cinnamon bark
clove
eucalyptus radiata
lemon
rosemary

Then add your favorite carrier oil such as olive oil.

NOTE: Clove and cinnamon bark are hot oils. So a carrier oil is recommended when applying them to your lips, face, or any sensitive skin areas to prevent a burning sensation.

*Mosquito Bites:*

Apply 1 to 2 drops of lavender or peppermint oil to any area where you've been bitten. Then to help keep the little "blood suckers" away, grab an empty small spray bottle and fill with 20 to 25 drops of the following oils:

cedarwood
citronella
lavender
lemongrass
peppermint

Fill the spray bottle with your favorite witch hazel you can buy at any drugstore, or places like Walgreens and Walmart (we recommend using organic witch hazel as it's healthier for your skin). Then spray on exposed skin areas as needed.

NOTE: Lavender essential oil is known to attract bees, so be cautious when using it while outside. You can eliminate lavender from this recipe if you're concerned about attracting bees.

*Perspiration (from Abby):*

Not too long ago I researched to see what was in traditional deodorant. Let me tell you, *I did not see that coming*!

It's really sad to see what people actually put in deodorant. There are many harmful chemicals in them, and I don't want them harming my body.

So I decided to do some experimenting by making my own deodorant. One day while practicing my dance for my recital, I was sweating because I was working really hard. But because I had used the deodorant I made, I didn't stink at all. I just smelled like coconut and citronella.

3 Tablespoons of cornstarch or arrowroot powder
1/2 teaspoon of sweet almond oil (optional)
2 heaping teaspoons of beeswax pellets
4 teaspoons of coconut oil
10 to 15 drops of your favorite essential oils (lavender, tea tree, or even citrus are some good choices, but it's up to you.)

First, fill a small pan a little less than halfway full of water and set it on the stove. Place a small glass bowl or container into the water, being careful not to get water in the bowl.

Place almond oil, beeswax and coconut oil in that same bowl or container. Then turn on the stove on medium heat, and allow the components to full melt.

Once they're fully melted, take the pan off of the stove and add your essential oils of choice, and cornstarch or arrowroot powder. Mix together until there are no clumps.

Carefully pour the mixture into a clean container, such as an old deodorant stick tube or even an old glue stick (they need to be really clean!) Allow it to cool, or put it in the fridge for at least 15 minutes until hardened.

Tada! You're done!

*Sunburns (from Abby)*

Have you ever heard of Myrrhmaid Lotion (this is one of my favorite recipes)? It protects your skin from harmful rays from the sun, while still allowing your body to get the vitamin SEA... um, I mean D... from the sun.

Apply 15 to 20 minutes before going into the pool so it doesn't wash off when you jump into the water. It's really easy to make, and you don't need very much.
organic unscented base lotion

an entire bottle of carrot seed essential oil
20 to 30 drops of myrrh essential oil
15 to 20 drops of lavender essential oil (optional)
a thin wooden dowel, or something to stir with

Unscrew the pump from your bottle of hand and body lotion. Then carefully pour the carrot seed oil into the bottle. Stir really well with the dowel. Or you can put the lid back on, then shake it really well.

Then you'll add the myrrh and lavender essential oils to the lotion. Once again, stir it all together with a dowel. Or put the lid on and shake it up. You can now put your pump back on and you're ready to apply to your skin.

Voila. You just made the perfect MyrrhMaid Lotion!

*Tired Feet:*

Do your feet hurt after wearing shoes all day (especially women who wear high heels)? Here's a recipe that will allow you to roll the aches away so you can enjoy wearing shoes 1 to 6 hours without any problems.

Drop the following essential oils into a 15ml (about 2.5 teaspoons) roller bottle (the kind that has a ball that rolls the liquid onto your skin):

20 to 25 drops of peppermint
20 to 25 drops of wintergreen
20 to 25 drops of copaiba
10 to 15 drops of lavender
5 to 10 drops of frankincense

Then fill the rest of the bottle with your favorite carrier oil such as olive oil. Reinstall your rollerball and lid.

Rolling on this new blend before and after wearing shoes (and throughout the day if it helps) can help ease tired, aching feet!

## Tips for Using Essential Oils Around Your Home

If you're looking for a more organic "green" way to get rid of harmful chemicals in your home, at work, and while you travel, you can make your own blend to use in a spray bottle to eliminate harmful toxins.

Use 100% plant and mineral-based oils such as lemon, clove, cinnamon bark, rosemary and eucalyptus. Not only will you get rid of nasty bacteria and toxins, your home will smell fabulous!

(You can also contact Jason about the special blend from the product line they use.)

## Body Soap (from Paige)

Here I'm going to teach you how to make BE-YOU-TIF-OIL soap!

Ingredients:

Your choice of essential oil for scent (i.e., lemon, eucalyptus, orange, rosemary, lavender, etc.)

7.5 ounces of white melt-n-pour soap (makes two bars). (This is a soap you melt in a pan on the stove, then pour into forms to create different shaped bars.)

food coloring (optional - we use fruit/veggie powders)
rubbing alcohol
microwave safe container
soap mold

First cut your soap into cubes. Then put the cubes into a microwave safe container, and microwave in 20-second bursts.

Take it out and stir well. If needed, you can put it back in the microwave for another 20-second burst. Once it's completely melted, add your oil(s) to the soap and stir well.

If you prefer to not use a microwave, fill a saucepan halfway with water. Place the glass jar with the soap into the water, and put the pan on the stove on medium heat. Allow the soap chunks to melt completely, then carefully remove the pan from the stove.

Using an oven mitt to protect yourself from getting burned, pour the soap from the jar into the mold and let it set for 40 minutes to 1 hour. Or you can put the mold into the refrigerator for 30 to 45 minutes.

After your soap has hardened, use your thumbs to pull aside the sides to release the suction. Then flip your mold over, and press down with your thumbs to release the soap. Not only will it smell beautiful, it's good for your skin, and can help your immune and respiratory systems.

## Dishwasher Detergent (from Paige)

It's important for my family to live toxin-free. So here I'm going to show you how to make your own essential oil dish detergent. (Since this is a powder soap, it's best used in a dishwasher, whereas a liquid detergent would be better for hand washing dishes. You could try to use this recipe for hand washing, but the powder would be harsh on your skin.)

1/2 cup baking soda
1/2 cup Borax soap
1/8 cup citric acid

Mix 10 drops each of the following essential oils together in a sealable container:

lemongrass
rosemary
your favorite citrus (lemon, orange, lime, etc.)
tea tree

Then add 1 Tablespoon to the water to have squeaky clean, sanitized, wonderfully smelling dishes (add an extra Tablespoon for heavy loads)!

## Fuzzy Bath Bombs (from Abby)

This is by far one of my favorite recipes. Making bath bombs is so much fun because you can make any scent you like in any size or shape.

1/3 cup of water
1 cup of organic baking soda
essential oils of your choice (I used 2 drops each of rosemary and lavender; then 3 drops peppermint, and 6 to 7 drops of eucalyptus)
small mixing bowl

Preheat your oven to 200 degrees.

Put the baking soda into a mixing bowl, then slowly add the water to make a sandy-like texture. Add the essential oils and stir together.

Roll the mixture into balls and place each one in a cup in a muffin tin. Be sure to use an oven-safe mold or pan to prevent the bath bombs from exploding or melting in your oven.

Once all the cups are filled, place them into in the oven for 40 to 45 minutes.

Put the muffin tin or mold on a rack, and allow the "bombs" to completely cool before putting into your bath water. You can also place one in the corner of your shower to make the water smell wonderful, and to benefit from inhaling the aroma!

*Soap Scrubs for Smooth Skin (from Abby)*

Today I figured out how to make soap scrubs. I've never actually used grated soap in my sugar scrubs, so this was a first.

This recipe is really easy and amazing. The scrub is very sweet and perfectly exfoliates your skin.

I decided to use lavender essential oil. The soap is an organic soap we buy from a vendor at our local farmer's market. But you can use any soap and essential oils you want. This recipe not only makes your kitchen smell so good as you're making it, it makes your skin feel fabulous!

a microwave-safe mixing bowl
a whisk
1/2 cup measuring cup
1/4 cup measuring cup
3/4 cup measuring cup
microwave oven
tablespoon for measuring
a mold you can put in the freezer (like a silicone mold you can get at almost any baking or cooking store)
a cheese grater

1/2 cup of your favorite soap (I used Eucalyptus Mint and Rosemary Sea Salt Goat Milk Soap from the soap company Soapize at the New Braunfels Farmers Market)
3/4 cup of organic pure cane sugar (make sure it's really grainy)
1/4 cup of organic olive oil
1 Tablespoon honey (optional)
dried flowers or herbs (optional)
your favorite essential oil(s) (I used lavender)

Grate your soap with a cheese grater until you have exactly one-half cup. Then pour the soap shavings into the mixing bowl. Add 1/4th cup of olive oil, then mix until combined.

Put the soap mixture into the microwave for 1 to 2 minutes at 10-second bursts just until the soap is completely melted (remember to use a microwavable container).

Add 3/4ths cup of sugar along with the honey and dried flowers or herbs. Then add the essential oil(s) of your choice. Mix until fully combined.

Now you're ready to pack the soaps into one or more molds, depending on their size. Make sure to really pack your scrub into the molds just like you were planting potting soil. Then stick the mold(s) into the freezer for 10 to 20 minutes until the soap is nice and hard.

*Springtime Flowers Sugar Scrub (from Abby)*

I've learned that the skin is the body's largest organ, and that everything you put in and on your body is important (which is why organic sugar and organic olive oil is recommended in this recipe).

I created then perfected this awesome sugar scrub recipe using all the springtime flowers you see everywhere in bloom. So I hope you try this recipe at home.

organic sugar
organic olive oil
geranium, hyssop, ylang ylang, lemon and lavender essential oils
1 small glass jar

First, fill the jar a little more than halfway full with organic sugar. Then add 3 to 4 Tablespoons of olive oil. Mix well until your scrub has the consistency of wet sand.

Then add 2 drops each of the following essential oils:

geranium
lemon
ylang ylang
hyssop
lavender

Mix together until well-combined. You might need to add more drops of oil until your scrub has the scent you desire.

## Aromatherapy Diffuser

Essential oils can be inhaled, added to drinks or food, or applied to your skin. One great to get the oil into the air is by using an aromatherapy diffuser as it's a simple, effective way to get the benefit of the oil while awake or asleep.

You can also get a car diffuser, and add peppermint and rosemary to keep you alert during long road trips or in bad traffic.

Another great way to use essential oils is through a product called the *Aromadome* (go to  aromadome.com for further information).

## Recipes Using Essential Oils

In his workbook, Ryan mentions the different kinds of issues that can benefit from the use of essential oils.

Many people don't realize that therapeutic grade essential oils can be used both topically and internally. Well, not all. But there are specific oils that can be used in smoothies and all sorts of recipes to help your body find balance and wellness.

Healthier diet plans – such as the Paleo diet – have taken the world by storm these past few years. People are trying to eliminate the toxins accumulated in their system from pollution, chemicals, and especially harmful medication.

There are thousands of recipes available on the Internet and in cookbooks. Following are just a few examples of how you can incorporate essential oils into food preparation:

*Banana Booster Bites (from Paige)*

1/2 cup almond butter
1/4 cup honey
2 cups oats
2 bananas
1 drop of cinnamon bark essential oil
2 Tablespoons of chocolate chips

Mix together. Then roll them into a ball and refrigerate. Enjoy your tasty treats!

*Fruit Smoothies*

There's nothing better than fresh fruit at their peak season from your garden, a farmer's market, or your local grocery store.

If your choices are slim, or aren't their optimum best, you can always use frozen fruit as their freshness is sealed tight. This way you can have them in your freezer year-round.

*Mango/Strawberry/Raspberry and Yogurt*

You could use any fruit combination. But these particular flavors work exceptionally well together.

1 scoop vanilla protein (the products the Sapps and Ryan use have an exceptional protein shake)
1/2 cup almond milk
1 cup frozen mango chunks
1/2 cup frozen strawberries
1/2 cup frozen raspberries
1/4 cup plain Greek yogurt
2 drops grapefruit essential oil
Toppings of your choice

Blend all ingredients, except toppings, together in a blender. If needed, add more milk or until mixture is smooth and not lumpy.

Separate into two bowls or tall glasses, and garnish with your choice of tasty toppings (i.e., sliced bananas, strawberries, almonds, walnuts, chia seeds, cherries, etc.).

*Spinach Pineapple*

1 cup unsweetened almond milk
3 cups baby spinach
1 cup fresh or frozen pineapple (not in cans as there's too much sugary syrup)
1 cup ice
2 drops of spearmint essential oil

Put ingredients in blender, then blend until smooth.

*Strawberry Watermelon*

1 cup unsweetened almond milk
1 cup frozen strawberries
1 cup watermelon
1 Tablespoon fresh basil
1 cup ice
1 to 3 drops of lemon essential oil

Put ingredients in blender, then blend until smooth.

## Lemonade

There's an old saying, "When life gets you down, make lemonade out of lemons."

Need a quick, cooling pick-me-up during those especially hot days? Use the following recipe to cool your body off internally, mentally and spiritually as well!

1 gallon glass jar with a dispenser tap
1-2 organic lemons
10-15 drops of lemon essential oil
Optional: add 1-3 drops of Lavender essential oil

Okay, so add water to just under the lid so you have room to stir. Then wash your lemons and slice. Then add them to your water. Put the lemon essential oils in as well as the optional lavender. Stir and taste. Adjust to your liking but we recommend starting with these drops and adding more to your liking because it is impossible to take out the drops once they are in your water!

## Pretty Perfect Parfait (from Paige)

Today I'll be teaching you how to make some Parfaits that are Pretty Perfect. This recipe is really fun and super easy:

2 boxes vanilla pudding
1-1/2 bananas and/or 1 kiwi
1/2 cup strawberries
1/2 cup blueberries
1 can mandarin oranges – drain off all liquid
2 cups milk
5 to 10 drops of orange essential oil
granola or graham crackers crushed to sprinkle on top or layered (optional, but they add a super yummy crunchiness1)

First pour milk and pudding powder in a small bowl. Stir for two minutes. Then add the orange essential oil and stir.

Next dice the strawberries and blueberries.

Layer pudding and each kind of fruit (according to photo) all the way to the top, including a layer of granola or graham crackers if you'd like. Top with graham cracker crumbs or granola and enjoy.

# Recap

Congratulations on taking a leap of faith toward overcoming your emotional, physical, psychological and spiritual healing! Our desire for anyone reading *The Miracle of Essential Oils* is that your prayers will be answered for a quick and painless recuperation. And that the information we've included on how to recognize your trauma, then overcome it with essential oils, can turn your life around faster than you ever thought possible.

Like receiving a birthday or Christmas gift, you first have to accept that you can heal. Then you can "unwrap" it to allow your healing. Having a balanced body can be a challenging task. But the efforts you put into finding balanced brain and body health will pay you many dividends.

As you continue to enter a new awareness, you might not know how to respond to situations, places and emotions that feel different or strange. While letting go of who you used to be, be grateful for all you're becoming with thanksgiving and joy in your heart. You can tackle anything that comes your way because you're now part of a growing community of essential oil users.

Our goal was to educate you on how to clear your emotions. You've been provided the list of emotions people with varying traumas typically tend to experience. But now you have the tools to overcome negative energetic emotions you might be struggling with.

Emotional healing comes in stages. Negative embedded emotions can be difficult to remove. So be patient with yourself, and diligently apply these different modalities with faith and intent.

If at all possible, don't go through this alone. Don't be afraid to ask for assistance, as your life is extremely valuable to you and your loved ones.

If it feels too difficult to accept your past, this might be a good time to seek professional help. Not all professionals are the same. Some are very traditional in their methods, while others are gifted and talented in the healing arts (or use a combination of both). For example, Ryan has worked with very talented pastors and lay individuals who possess the gift of healing therapy. So finding a therapist who specializes in this particular area of trauma can help you grow and change.

Before we wrap this up, we'd like you to answer a few questions to determine how well you've absorbed this information:

When did you start your journey to healing your trauma or difficulty?

_____

What changes did you expect before you began your journey?

_____
_____
_____

What changes have you seen in yourself while working through the information in this book?

_____
_____
_____

In your honest opinion, how hard have you worked to have positive changes?

_____
_____
_____

What are your expectations in moving forward?

_____
_____
_____

How will you know when you've met these expectations?

_____
_____
_____

Are you open to discussing with others the changes you're experiencing? _____ Yes _____ No

If yes, don't hesitate to contact Jason or Ryan with any questions or concerns.

**_Remember, you don't have to go through this alone!_**

We hope you'll be eternally grateful for all that has been done and will continue to be done on your behalf. There are people like us who understand what you've gone through. All you have to take is take the first step to reach out then allow them to help.

Writing this book was more than a labor of purpose – it was a labor of love. Our goal with sharing what we've learned about essentials oils was to empower you to find answers to your healing, and to life without pain. So hopefully we've achieved that and much more.

We ask that you to pay it forward by sharing this book and its message with others to help them overcome their struggles. Maybe all it takes is one word, one paragraph, or one chapter to begin their own journey to wellness.

Once you begin to see the oils' many benefits, we'd love you to share your experiences (and this book) with others who might be dealing with issues where these oils can bring relief. (We'd also love you to send us your testimonials via our email listed at the end of book.)

To those of you serving in the military, God bless you and your family for all of the sacrifices and selfless services you made for our country. To the rest of you, may abundant blessings be bestowed upon you and your family from this day forward.

*Ryan Watson, M. Ed. and Jason Sapp*

# References

*Articles and Books:*

Alcoholics Anonymous Big Book (2007). Alcoholics Anonymous (AA) World Services.

Amen, Dr. Daniel G. (2015): *Change Your Brain, Change Your Life (Revised and Expanded): The Breakthrough Program for Conquering Anxiety, Depression, Obsessiveness, Lack of Focus, Anger, and Memory Problems.* Harmony Publishers

American Psychiatric Association (2013). *Diagnostic and Statistical Manual of Mental Disorders* (5th ed.). Arlington, VA: American Psychiatric Publishing.

Becker, Dr. Robert O. (1998). *The Body Electric: Electromagnetism and the Foundation of Life.* William Morrow; 1st Quill Ed edition.

Brown, Brené (August, 2010): *Gifts of Imperfection.* Hazelden Publishing; 1st edition.

Burk, Arthur and Sylvia Gunter (2009): *Blessing Your Spirit.* Plumbline Ministries.

Burroughs, Stanley (1993). *Healing for the Age of Enlightenment.* Burroughs Books.

Carelli. R. M. (2002): *The Nucleus Accumbens and Reward: Neurophysiological Investigations in Behaving Animals.* Behavioral Cognitive Neuroscience.

Demos, John N. (2005). *Getting Started With Neurofeedback.* W.W. Norton & Company, New York.

Essential Oils Desk Reference (March 2004). Essential Science Publishing; 3rd edition.

Fisher, Sebern F. (2014). *Neurofeedback in the Treatment of Developmental Trauma: Calming the Fear-Driven Brain.* New York City. W.W. Norton & Company.

Foster, Dale S, Robert W. Thatcher (2015): "Surface and LORETA Neurofeedback in the Treatment of Post-Traumatic Stress Disorder and Mild Traumatic Brain Injury." Science Direct.

Gattefossé, R. M., and R. B. Tisserand (ed.) (1993). *Gattefossé's Aromatherapy: The First Book on Aromatherapy.* C. W. Daniel, Saffron Walden.

Hay, Louise (1988). *Heal Your Body.* Hay House. Carlsbad, California.

*How Many Calories Are Actually in Your Salad?* Huffington Post. February 20, 2013.

Hyman, Dr. Mark. (30 December, 2014): *The Blood Sugar Solution.* Little, Brown and Company; Reprint edition.

Koderba, J. L. (2014). *Z-score LORETA Neurofeedback as a Potential Therapy in Depression/Anxiety and Cognitive Dysfunction.* Academic Press, San Diego, CA.

Lawlis, Frank (2010). *The PTSD Breakthrough.* Sourcebooks, Illinois.

Mein, D.C., Carolyn L. (1998). *Releasing Emotional Patterns with Essential Oils.* Vision Ware Press, California. (See URL below for *The Script*)

Milkman, H. and S. Sunderwith (2010). *Cravings for Ecstasy and Natural Highs.* Sage Press.

Nelson, Dr. Bradley (2007): *The Emotion Code.* Wellness Unmasked Publishing.

New King James Version Bible. Harper Collins. 1982.

New International Version Bible. Biblica. 2011.

Oschman, James L. (2000). *Energy Medicine.* Churchill Livingstone Press.

Raine, Adrian (2014): *The Anatomy of Violence: The Biological Roots of Crime.* Vintage Press.

Raybern, Debra, Sera Johnson, Laura and Karen Hopkins (2008). *Nutrition 101: Choose Life!* Growing Health Homes.

Stewart, David (2003). *Healing Oils of the Bible.* Care Publications, Missouri.

Stewart, David (2010). *The Chemistry of Essential Oils.* CARE Publications, Missouri.

Tennant, Jerry L. (2013). *Healing is Voltage, Cancer's On/Off Switches: Polarity.* Create Space Independent Publishing Platform.

Trimm, Cindy (2007). *Commanding Your Morning: Unleashing The Power of God in Your Life.* Charisma House, Lake Mary Florida.

Truman, Karol K. (1991). *Feelings Buried Alive Never Die.* Olympus Distributing.

Tyrrell, Michael. (2014). *WholeTones: The Sound of Healing.* Barton Publishing, Brandon, SD.

Wright, Pastor Henry (2009). *A More Excellent Way.* Whitaker House.

Young, D. Gary (2013). *Essential Oils Integrative Medical Guide.* Life Science Publishing, Utah.

*Websites:*

Allen, Dr. Corinne. *Light Beyond Trauma.* DVD
http://www.discoverlsp.com/multimedia/light-beyond-trauma-dvd-set-4.html

Allen, Dr. Corinne. *The Script.* Brain Advance.
http://brainadvance.org/

*Aromatherapy in the Workplace.* Editorial. Personnel Today.
http://www.personneltoday.com/hr/aromatherapy-in-the-workplace

Bible References for Essential Oils.
http://www.keepsmilin.com/bblref.html

Bonds-Garrett, Dr. Christi. Vibrational Raindrop Method.
http://www.drbondsgarrett.com/

Bonnell, Gwenn. Tap into Heaven.
http://www.tapintoheaven.com/index_welcome.shtml

*Causes of Symptoms According to Louise Hay.* The Alchemy of Healing.
http://alchemyofhealing.com/causes-of-symptoms-according-to-louise-hay/

Church, Dr. Dawson. *EFT Tapping: Dawson Church PhD Introduces Emotional Freedom Techniques.*
http://www.youtube.com/watch?v=77BY5LzW36A

Church, Dr. Dawson. *The Veteran's Stress Project.*
http://stressproject.org/

*Diagnostic and Statistical Manual of Mental Disorders.* Fifth Edition. Psychiatry Online.
http://dsm.psychiatryonline.org/doi/book/10.1176/appi.books.97808 90425596

Diamond, Dr. John (editorial): Behavioral Kinesiology: A Different Procedure.
http://www.drjohndiamond.com/papers/106-behavioral-kinesiology-a-different-procedure

Doward, James (8 February, 2014). Organic Food Back in Vogue as Sales Increase.
http://www.theguardian.com/environment/2014/feb/09/organic-produce-sales-increase

Emoto, Masuru. What is the Photograph of Frozen Water Crystals?
http://www.masaru-emoto.net/english/water-crystal.html

Fight-or-Flight-Response. Wikipedia.
http://en.wikipedia.org/wiki/Fight-or-flight_response

Friedmann, Terry (2001): *Attention Deficit and Hyperactivity Disorder (ADHD).*
http://files.meetup.com/1481956/ADHD%20Research%20by%20Dr.% 20Terry%20Friedmann.pdf

Hara, Dr. Carmen (6 July, 2013). *35 Affirmations That Will Change Your Life.*
http://huffingtonpost.com

Hawkins, David R.
http://www.veritaspub.com/

Heart Math.
http://www.heartmath.com

Hecht, Steven (2005): Re. Dr. John Zimmerman. "The Era of Energy Medicine." *Spirit of Change* Magazine.
http://www.spiritofchange.org/May-June-2005/The-Era-of-Energy-Medicine/

History of Neuroplasticity.
http://www.whatisneuroplasticity.com/history.php

*How Many Calories Are in Your Salad?* (20 February, 2013). The
Huffington Post.
http://www.huffingtonpost.com/2014/08/11/portion-sizes-salad-
calories-ingredients_n_2719726.html

Journal of Essential Oil Research. November, 2014. Issue 2.
http://www.tandfonline.com/toc/tjeo20/current

Lewis, Jordan Gaines, Ph.D. (12 January, 2015): *Smells Ring Bells:
How Smell Triggers Memories and Emotions.*
http://www.psychologytoday.com/blog/brain-babble/201501/smells-
ring-bells-how-smell-triggers-memories-and-emotions

Kirlian Photography.
http://en.wikipedia.org/wiki/Kirlian_photography

Koberda, J. Lucas (2015): "Z-score LORETA Neurofeedback as a
Potential Therapy in Depression/Anxiety and Cognitive Dysfunction.
Science Direct."
http://www.sciencedirect.com/science/article/pii/B97801280129180
00054

Korotkov, Dr. Konstantin: The Biowell Imaging Machine
http://www.korotkov.eu/

MedlinePlus
http://www.medlineplus.gov

Mein, Dr. Caroline. "Clearing Emotional Patterns" (download).
http://www.wildessentialoils.com/pdf/releasing-emotional-
patterns.pdf

Nagpal, M.L., K. Gleichauf and J.P. Ginsberg (2013):  Study: A Meta-
Analysis of Heart Rate Variability as a Psychophysiological Indicator of
Posttraumatic Stress Disorder.
http://www.omicsgroup.org/journals/metaanalysis-of-heart-rate-
variability-as-a-psychophysiological-indicator-of-posttraumatic-stress-
disorder-2167-1222.1000182.pdf

National Center for PTSD (U.S. Department of Veterans Affairs)
http://www.ncptsd.va.gov/

National Institute of Mental Health (NIMH)
http://www.nimh.nih.gov

National Institute of Neurological Disorders and Stroke
http://www.ninds.nih.gov

Paradigm
http://https://en.wikipedia.org/wiki/Paradigm

"Post-Traumatic Stress Disorder" (editorial)
http://www.military.com/benefits/veterans-health-care/posttraumatic-stress-disorder-overview.html

Post-Traumatic Stress Disorder. The Nebraska Department of Veterans'
Affairs.
http://www.ptsd.ne.gov/what-is-ptsd.html

Reams, Dr. Carey. The Advanced Ideals Institute (RBTI).
http://www.advancedideals.org/01_who_we_are.html and
http://newtreatments.org/reams

Sayorwan, W., et al (23 December, 2012): "Effects of
inhaled rosemary oil on subjective feelings and activities of the nervous
system." National Center for Biotechnology Information (NCBI).
http://www.ncbi.nlm.nih.gov/pubmed/?term=Rosemary+and+beta+waves

Suicide Data Report (2012). Department of Veterans Affairs Mental
Health Services Suicide Prevention Program.
http://www.va.gov/opa/docs/suicide-data-report-2012-final.pdf

Suicide in the United States
http://en.wikipedia.org/wiki/Suicide

Tainio, Bruce. "Vibrational Frequency and the Subtle Energy Nature of
Essential Oils."
http://www.biospiritual-energy-healing.com/vibrational-frequency.html

Taub Therapy Clinic: Get Back What Your Stroke Took Away
http://taubtherapy.com/index.php?pid=9795

The Tapping Solution
http://www.thetappingsolution.com/what-is-eft-tapping/

Trauma Release Script
http://www.brainadvance.org/trauma___block_release_script

Trauma Screening Questionnaire: National Center for PTSD (Veterans Administration).
http://www.ptsd.va.gov/professional/assessment/screens/tsq.asp

23andMe Genetic Diagnostics
https://www.23andme.com/

*Types of Trauma and Violence* (editorial). Substance Abuse and Mental Health Administration (SAMHSA).
http://www.samhsa.gov/trauma-violence/types

United States Military Veteran Suicide
http://en.wikipedia.org/wiki/United_States_military_veteran_suicide

Voris, John. (3 July, 2009): *The Difference Between Emotions and Feelings.*
http://johnvoris.com/featured-articles/difference-between-emotions-and-feelings/

Weil, Dr. Andrew. *Applied Kinesiology.* Well Therapies.
http://www.drweil.com/drw/u/ART03410/Applied-Kinesiology.html

Wilson, Dr. Ralph. In his video at http://www.youtube.com/watch?v=7StVJAkctZU, Dr. Wilson illustrates the teeth and the acumeridians tooth relationship. For further information, you can visit his website at www.integrativehomeopathy.com.

# About the Authors

## RYAN WATSON, M.ED.

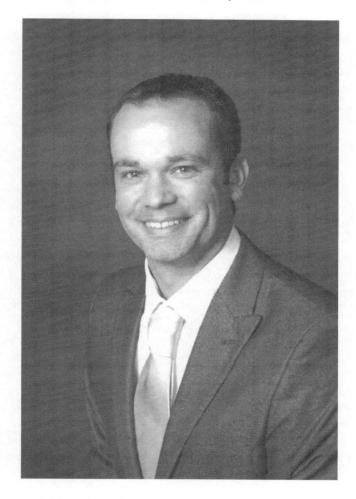

The director and founder of the Watson Psychological Health Center in Amarillo, Texas, Ryan Watson graduated from Texas Tech University with a Master's in Educational Psychology.

His professional training include the areas of:

- Biofeedback
- Biological Analysis
- Brain Integration
- Clinical Hypnotherapy
- Emotional Release Techniques
- Eye Movement Desensitization and Reprocessing (EMDR)

- Heart Rate Variability
- Meditation
- Neurofeedback

Ryan has worked in a therapeutic setting for over a decade assisting individuals of all ages. He specializes in:

- ADD, ADHD
- Adolescent issues
- Anger and control issues
- Depression, stress and anxiety
- Many levels of addictions
- Marital and relationship issues
- Trauma and PTSD

An author, educator and professional speaker, Ryan often speaks to large audiences on specialized topics of mental health and the neural developmental aspects of behavior.

In 2012, he opened the Watson Psychological Health Center (WPHC) to focus on the advancement of neurofeedback. WPHC – that offers modalities that aren't commonly available in many areas of Texas – incorporates scientific data about the brain and body into a client's treatments.

WPHC provides the following services:

- Neurofeedback / Biofeedback
- Eye Movement Desensitization and Reprocessing (EMDR)
- Biological Analysis
- The Reconnect Intensive Program
- The Marriage Intensive Program
- Smoking Cessation and Addiction Treatment
- Online Services

Ryan has created intensive four-day programs where he works with individuals or couples each day based on their needs. His beautiful, tranquil location allows their progress in a very unique way.

To contact him about any of these services – or if there's something you would like to discuss that's not on the list – you can contact him via the sources below:

Website: www.watsonphc.com/
Email: info@watsonphc.com

# JASON SAPP

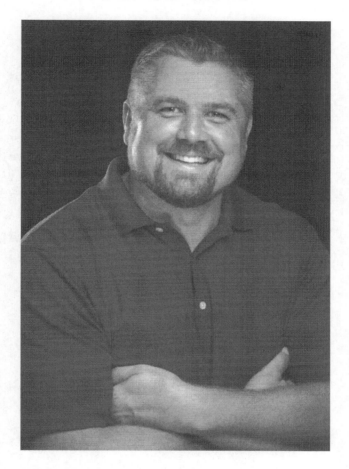

My goal after being honorably discharged from the U.S. Army was to go to college and earn a degree. I finally accomplished this in December, 2015, when I graduated from Liberty University with a BS in Business Administration in Entrepreneurship.

While I and my wife, La'Nette, are building our essential oil and aromatherapy business, I'm working toward a Masters of Divinity in Theology from Liberty University.

To contact Jason and La'Nette about their essential oil and aromatherapy products, training sessions and any upcoming seminars and special events:

Website: www.essentoilyblessed.com

Email: TheSapps@essentoilyblessed.com
Facebook: http://www.facebook.com/LaNetteSapp?fref=ts

To get on Jason's list to let you know when *The Battle Within* has been launched, send him a note via sgtjasonsapp@yahoo.com. Or sign up for his email list at thebattle-within.com.

* * * * * * *

We encourage you to Like and follow us on our Facebook page at http://www.facebook.com/paradigmpress as we'll be providing training events and live Q&As on a regular basis.

Make sure to bookmark our website paradigmpressshop.com as well to find out about events and speaking engagements. If you have any questions about the content of this book, or where to purchase additional copies, you can contact us via paradigmpressllc@gmail.com, or paradigmpressshop.com.

If you've like us to speak at one of your events, you can contact us by email at paradigmpressllc@gmail.com for information and availability.

51811282R00127

Made in the USA
Lexington, KY
06 September 2019